FAMILY THERAPY THEORY FOR NURSING

FOUR APPROACHES

FAMILY THERAPY THEORY FOR NURSING

FOUR APPROACHES

Ann L. Whall, Ph.D., F.A.A.N.
Professor
University of Michigan
School of Nursing
Ann Arbor, Michigan

APPLETON-CENTURY-CROFTS/Norwalk, Connecticut

0-8385-2549-0

Notice: The author(s) and publisher of this volume have taken care that the information and recommendations contained herein are accurate and compatible with the standards generally accepted at the time of publication.

86 87 88 89 90 / 10 9 8 7 6 5 4 3 2 1

Prentice-Hall of Australia, Pty. Ltd., Sydney
Prentice-Hall Canada, Inc.
Prentice-Hall Hispanoamericana, S.A., Mexico
Prentice-Hall of India Private Limited, New Delhi
Prentice-Hall International (UK) Limited, London
Prentice-Hall of Japan, Inc., Tokyo
Prentice-Hall of Southeast Asia (Pte.) Ltd., Singapore
Whitehall Books Ltd., Wellington, New Zealand
Editora Prentice-Hall do Brasil Ltda., Rio de Janeiro

Library of Congress Cataloging-in-Publication Data

Family therapy theory for nursing.

1. Family psychotherapy. 2. Psychiatric nursing.
I. Whall, Ann L. [DNLM: 1. Family Therapy—methods.
2. Psychiatric Nursing—methods. WY 160 F1986]
RC488.5.F353 1986 616.89'156 86-17449
ISBN 0-8385-2549-0

Design: M. Chandler Martylewski
Cover: Cindy Lee Lombardo

PRINTED IN THE UNITED STATES OF AMERICA

Contributors

Carol Boyd, M.S.N., R.N., F.A.A.N.
Doctoral Candidate
Wayne State University
College of Nursing
Detroit, Michigan

Paula W. Gonot, Ph.D., R.N.
Vice President
Nursing Systems
Grant Medical Center
and
Adjunct Assistant Professor
College of Nursing
The Ohio State University
Columbus, Ohio

Ruth L. Johnston, Ph.D., R.N.
Consultant in Geropsychiatric Nursing
Clinical Nurse Specialist in Psychiatric Mental Health
Gresham, Oregon

Susan L. Jones, Ph.D., R.N., C.S.
Professor
Kent State University
School of Nursing
Kent, Ohio

Pamela G. Reed, Ph.D., R.N.
Assistant Professor
University of Arizona
School of Nursing
Tucson, Arizona

Jean A. Werner-Beland, M.N., R.N., C.S., F.A.A.N.
Rehabilitation Counselor
Clinical Nurse Specialist in Psychiatric Mental Health
North Port, Florida

Ann L. Whall, Ph.,D., F.A.A.N.
Professor
University of Michigan
School of Nursing
Ann Arbor, Michigan

Ann M. Zuzich, M.S.N., R.N.
Associate Professor
Wayne State University
College of Nursing
Detroit, Michigan

Contents

Preface

Of the many new trends in nursing today, one of the most exciting is the current emphasis upon advanced practice. This area has not, however, been related to a great degree to theory development efforts in nursing. That is, in my experience, graduate theory development courses are often not specifically related to advanced practice approaches. Although students are expected to synthesize these two areas of content, this goal of synthesis is difficult to meet because few texts are available that specifically relate theory development efforts and practice. Theory development texts, moreover, do not usually delve at any length into specific practice approaches. This text is designed to redress the separation of advanced practice and theory development in the practice area of family therapy.

Family therapy is by now accepted as an advanced practice area for nursing. Family therapy theories, however, have been for the most part developed outside of nursing. These existing theories frequently prescribe activities that I believe are not consistent with the perspective of nursing as articulated in the Standard of Practice, the Social Policy Statement, and nursing models. If nursing is to develop a cohesive body of knowledge upon which to base practice, it is counterproductive to our efforts to use without change theories from other disciplines that are not consistent with the perspective of nursing. The purpose of this text is, therefore, to assist in the development of nursing knowledge in the area of family therapy by demonstrating ways in which the theoretical base for practice might be further developed.

The theoretical approaches presented in each chapter are not finished attempts by any means, in fact they may be viewed as partial theory or approaches which need to be further developed in terms of concepts and relationships. To wait to present these approaches until they are well developed would, I believe, delay the needed discussions. In the view of this text, nursing models may be used to develop family therapy approaches. It is also shown to be important to recognize that nurses who practice family therapy develop expert knowledge which may then be articulated as specific nursing approaches to family therapy. These two types of knowledge can be used to further develop theory for practice as well as to examine theories outside of nursing for relevance to and reformulation of the discipline.

Questions of whether the approaches presented in this text are better than approaches currently existing outside of nursing are premature and rather miss the point that nursing needs to develop theory supportive of and consistent with its practice goals. Also, determination of "better" depends on the viewpoint from which one is judging. Because each theory describes family health differently, "better" outcomes for one theory may not be "better" outcomes for another theory.

The many excellent nursing theory texts published yearly have diminished arguments over which is the "one way" to proceed to develop a comprehensive body of nursing knowledge. There is recognition now that many approaches to theory development have merit. There is little discussion, however, as to the multiple ways one might develop specific nursing knowledge for the practice of family therapy.

In an earlier text, *Nursing Models and Their Psychiatric Mental Health Applications*, I began the discussion of ways in which a nursing approach to family therapy might be developed. This present text may be viewed as an extension of that earlier work. In the first text a comparative analysis and reformulation was made with the purpose of reformulating psychiatric mental health theories using nursing models for the reformulation. The present text is also concerned with reformulation; however, nursing models are used not only to examine and reformulate existing theory but also to derive psychiatric mental health nursing approaches. In addition, nursing knowledge that has been developed inductively through the practice experiences of nurse family therapists is used to reformulate existing theory from outside the discipline.

The present text is an effort, therefore, to present to graduate students as well as to practitioners specific nursing approaches to family therapy. Undergraduates may also find this text helpful in working with families, although undergraduates would not conduct family therapy per se. Rather than focusing primarily upon theory building techniques themselves, this text addresses the development of four basic concepts: *family, family health, family environment*, and *nurse therapist*, in the therapy approaches presented. By focusing upon these four concepts the authors present distinctive nursing approaches to family therapy. Each author is a psychiatric clinical nurse specialist with much experience in dealing with families in therapy. Each brings to her chapter this experiential base. Recognition is given to nurse theorists King, Roy, and Rogers, who assisted in the interpretation of their models for specific chapters of this text; their assistance was most helpful. This text was written, revised, and rewritten over the past three years and through these efforts the authors have clarified their ideas. It is our hope that this work will inspire others to thoughtfully examine the ways in which theoretical bases for nursing practice differ from and are similar to those of other disciplines. In this way the theoretical bases for advanced clinical practice will continue to be developed. Nursing has made great progress in the last few years toward developing this type of knowledge. The future appears promising and the fulfillment of the goal of developing a comprehensive knowledge base for our specific advanced practice areas appears to be at hand.

Ann L. Whall

FAMILY THERAPY THEORY FOR NURSING

FOUR APPROACHES

1

Introduction: Theoretical Perspectives

Ann L. Whall

Nursing is in the midst of an exciting new era, one in which theory development issues are generally understood, and one in which advanced nursing practice is well established. The merging of these two trends makes possible stimulating new discussions of the ways to structure knowledge for this advanced practice. These discussions need to be articulated so that various approaches to this knowledge development may be debated and evaluated. In addition, the practice knowledge generated by these various approaches needs to be presented and examined. These then are the two purposes of this text, first to present four methods by which knowledge may be developed for an advanced practice area in nursing, that of family therapy, and secondly to present examples of these development efforts.

Chapter 1 presents an explanation of the four development approaches. Chapters 2 through 8 present examples of ways in which these efforts might be developed. These examples are not finished attempts by any means; rather, they are a beginning attempt for further practice examination and explication. Before beginning these discussions, however, the term *family therapy* as used to describe an advanced nursing practice area must be defined.

The term *therapy* has taken on, to some, the meaning of pathology or the connotation of a mechanic operating upon the mental functioning of family members. In this text the term therapy is used in its original sense, from the Greek *therapeutikos* meaning "attendant." Nurses attend for the most part families who are experiencing a troubling situation. The emphasis is, therefore, upon "working with" rather than "operating upon" families, which is consistent with nursing's heritage and its emphasis upon the self-assessment of the nurse and mutual goal setting. The nursing approach thus implies a "working with" rather than an "operating upon" families. The major assumptions upon which this text is based are discussed below.

THE BACKGROUND

Before proceeding with this important exploration, a few assumptions must be identified. One such assumption is that each discipline is responsible for developing and examining its own knowledge base, and that in the case of a professional discipline such as nursing, this creation and examination are essential because the service rendered to society is predicated upon this knowledge.

Johnson (1974) long ago discussed the need for development of a distinct body of theoretical knowledge for nursing. She stated, "If nursing is indeed an emerging profession, nurses must be able to identify clearly and develop continually the theoretical body of knowledge upon which practice must rest" (p. 372). Ellis (1968) referred to the need for a distinct body of knowledge when she discussed the need to synthesize content from diverse fields for nursing. Fawcett (1983) discussed the need for nursing to develop its own knowledge base if it is to be considered a legitimate discipline. Knowledge within a discipline, therefore, needs to be developed from the perspective of that discipline, in this case, nursing.

Donaldson and Crowley (1978) addressed the difference between academic and professional disciplines in terms of clarification of relationships in academe. They discussed that disciplines are not built upon each other in a Chinese box fashion, but rather that each discipline develops its own knowledge base, related but distinct from another. Nursing practice in this view must be based upon knowledge developed for the discipline. Another assumption of this text is that if nurse–practitioners are to work in a therapeutic capacity with families, it is essential that they systematically develop the knowledge upon which they base their practice and that they not only continue to examine this knowledge but remain aware of theoretical issues involved.

These assumptions are not considered attempts toward territoriality because professional disciplines are mandated by society to carry out certain activities. Without the properly developed and verified knowledge upon which to base these activities, the mandate cannot be adequately fulfilled. Because nursing has different goals as well as different societal mandates than medicine, for example, its approaches are different. Nursing needs to continue to develop its own knowledge base, drawing upon existing knowledge from other disciplines where appropriate. Kaplan (1963) addressed the latter situation, of interaction between disciplines, when he stated that some of the most exciting encounters in the history of science occur when two distinct fields are brought together.

Another assumption upon which this text is based is that knowledge is developed in a variety of ways, and that each method has advantages as well as disadvantages. Indeed, multiple theory development strategies for nursing are currently being discussed and debated (Meleis, 1985). It is believed that multiple methods should be used to develop knowledge for the discipline and that those developing this knowledge should be aware of the problems that are inherent in each method. Two major methods that have been discussed are deductive processes (from the abstract to the more specific level), inductive processes (from the particular to the more general), and, in addition, borrowing and reformulating. When borrowing knowledge it is important that the borrowed knowledge be changed so as to fit the perspective of nursing.

FOUR APPROACHES USED IN THIS TEXT

One may develop family therapy theory for nursing by deductively deriving an approach from a nursing model, such as that of Rogers (1970, 1980). Conceptual models are distinguished from theoretical models or theories in large part on the basis of level of abstraction, the conceptual models being the more abstract (Fawcett, 1978). Fawcett identified other differences between theories and conceptual models (e.g., the concepts or terms contained in a conceptual model are often broad and multidimensional). Theories, on the other hand, have concepts that are more specific. In addition, the interrelationships between concepts in conceptual models are often not as explicit as those found in theories. Conceptual models are thus broad umbrellas from which theories may be derived or developed. Rogers' conceptual model in this view is not at a theoretical level, but may be used for the development of many theories.

There are at the present time few theories in nursing that have been developed from nursing models. Nursing models are available, however, for this development and may be used to deductively derive middle-range or micro-level theories or to reformulate existing theories. What must be addressed when deriving a theoretical approach to families from these models, however, is the systematic examination of the models in terms of discussion of family. Clements and Roberts (1983) have facilitated this effort by presenting several nurse–theorists' discussions of the ways in which their models are applicable to families. Family therapy, however, is not described by Clements' and Roberts' discussion nor is it their purpose.

One of the problems in terms of either the deductive development of family theory from a nursing model or of reformulating existing theory using a nursing model concerns the level of abstraction found within nursing models. If an approach to the family is to be derived from these models, a good deal of inference must be used. It would follow that the derivations, even if consistent and congruent with the model, would be quite different depending upon the individual interpretation. Although this is a problem, it should be recognized that nurses currently use conceptual models from other disciplines and make the necessary conceptual leaps and thereby draw individual inferences upon which they base their practice. In other words, a major difference would be the use of a nursing model as opposed to use of a conceptual model outside of nursing. It must be stressed that all inferences drawn and approaches derived should be subject to empirical verification through research, practice examination, or both. Research and other scientific examination of tentative theoretical statements have always been accepted and needed steps in all theory development efforts.

One advantage in using the nursing models to derive practice knowledge is that the models are often well known and accepted in nursing and that the models address essential elements with which nursing is concerned. Because most advanced nursing practice programs provide courses that familiarize students with the nursing models, the availability of the models and the familiarity of students with the models makes them an important resource for the development of practice approaches. Kaplan (1963) has addressed advantages inherent in the use of models in theory building efforts (e.g., complex phenomena may be handled simply in models). In the case of the nursing models, the complex phenomenon "person" is often characterized quite simply as a "bio/psycho/social being." Another advantage Kaplan identified in using models is that gaps in knowledge are more easily identified. For example, because conceptual models are broad abstractions which may encompass several more specific theories, models often indicate areas of theory building that have been overlooked by more specific theories, and also indicate concepts and relationships that need to be further examined. Areas where more work is needed to specifically identify relationships for a nursing approach to family therapy may therefore be identified when nursing models are used, and the models may therefore lead to new questions about a nursing approach to family therapy.

Deductive and Inductive Approaches

As can be seen in the Summary, there are two general approaches used to develop family therapy knowledge for nursing: the deductive approach and the inductive approach. These approaches are further divided into two types of deductive strategies and two types of inductive strategies. In the two deductive strategies, nursing models are used to either derive a family therapy approach using deductive inference or to deduce approaches that would change an existing therapy theory so as to be consistent with the nursing model. In two inductive approaches found in this text, empirical relationships are stated about specific situations and then are used as a guide for changing existing therapy theory. The last chapter in this text is not based upon any one existing theory but rather on an approach inductively developed by Zuzich through experience over her years of work with families.

As with the deductive approaches, there are advantages and disadvantages to the inductive approach. The advantages according to Maslow (1966) are that experiential knowledge expands rather than weakens the empirical attitude. That is, an empirical process is an effort to unify experiential knowledge so that a new whole may be perceived (Maslow, 1966).

One disadvantage to the inductive approach, according to Maslow, is that it is easy to carry a simple truth beyond its proper limits. In other words, when going from the specific to the general, the logic may not hold. Popper (1968) discussed that one cannot infer that all swans are white because one has only observed white swans. Perhaps one way to counteract this problem is not to make too great a claim for one's personal observations. In other words, to identify that other possibilities exist but that in many cases the inductively derived knowledge will be useful.

There are two ways in which existing theories are used in this text: these borrowed theories are either changed, using knowledge deduced from a nursing model, or they are reformulated, using nursing knowledge inductively developed in nursing practice. In the view of this text it is necessary to change these theories borrowed from outside the discipline so as to fit the perspective of nursing. Nonreformulation is considered an error with serious consequences for nursing if one believes in the necessity for each discipline to develop the theoretical base to carry out its societal mandate (Whall, 1980).

Family therapy theories developed outside nursing are at a more specific or less abstract level than the nursing models. Consequently, the reformulation attempts using a nursing model are referred to as deductive reformulation, or deriving knowledge deductively from a nursing model, and then this viewpoint is used to address and change major aspects of the existing family therapy theory. When the attempt at reformulation is approached using inductively derived nursing knowledge, the reformulation is termed inductive reformulation.

The general format used for each chapter is the same although the authors developed their chapter in a manner suited to their needs. Each contributor was asked to identify the way in which the four central concepts of nursing might be handled in each of the approaches found in this text (i.e., the deductive, the inductive, the borrowed theory deductively reformulated, and the borrowed theory inductively reformulated). Rather than handling the four central concepts as they are (i.e., person, environment, health, and nursing) the concepts were generally reconceptualized as family, family environment, family health, and the therapist's approach or the healing process. This is a logical step because therapists, for the most part, consider the family as a unit, not just as individual persons within the family. Further, the family environment external to the family has always been considered important in nursing, although this is not always the case with other disciplines (Whall, 1982). Family health, or the optimal state which is the goal of nursing, is addressed either implicitly or explicitly as nurses interact with families. Nursing, as the verb or the active component of the four concepts, is in this text identified in terms of the nurse–therapist. In this regard, the therapeutic process itself is described and developed by each author with a practice example.

One final issue, the graduate level preparation in family therapy which exists in psychiatric mental health nursing programs across the United States, is seen as necessary preparation for nurses who practice family therapy. This preparation is mandated by the Psychiatric Mental Health Nursing Standards of Practice. Along with supervised therapy experience, this background prepares nurses for practice in this field. In the author's experience, family therapy is practiced at a mental health nursing clinic controlled and staffed by faculty and students in a university setting. In this mental health nursing clinic (MHNC), faculty who work with individuals, families, and groups and also practice, use either inductively derived or deductively derived nursing approaches. At the MHNC, this author uses a deductive reformulated approach, one example of which is presented in Chapter 4. This clinic is described in more detail elsewhere (Whall, 1985). The work of Andersen (1982) describes an approach used at MHNC that was deductively derived from Rogers' (1970, 1980) conceptual model. Andersen's approach is not specifically addressed in this text because it applies to individual therapy.

In terms of the above discussion, Schwab (1964) discussed science as being in essence a process of constructing bodies of tentative knowledge and of discovering different ways of making data coherent. This text is an attempt to demonstrate ways in which nursing knowledge may be developed for the practice of family therapy and, in a sense, to make family data coherent for the nurse-practitioner. This is an exciting time in nursing, wherein various approaches to practice knowledge may be proposed, debated, refined, and revised. This text is presented in that spirit. The examples in chapters 2 through 8 are not finished attempts and the reader is invited to explore, debate, and revise these beginning efforts. In this way, nursing will continue to construct tentative knowledge and to search for various ways of developing the much needed theoretical base.

At the outset, it was recognized that the term *family* needed to be clarified. Perhaps the term family can be best understood by the following. When families present themselves for assistance they define for themselves who is their family. The concept "family" to them may mean anything from "a married pair with dependent children" to "a group of individuals who join together to support and assist one another sometimes for a specific purpose" (Butler & Lewis, 1982, p. 150). Thus persons presenting themselves to the nurse for assistance will define for themselves who is their family. Those persons will care little for objective definitions of "family," for to them it has a very personal meaning. In that the nurse begins by working with persons who present themselves as a family, the family's definition will need to suffice. The nurse–therapist, therefore, must live with a certain amount of ambiguity in terms of the definition of the concept "family." As far as the nursing models and the inductive approaches are concerned, each theoretical approach defines the family in slightly different ways. The author of each chapter was asked to address the way the concept "family" as a unit is discussed in each approach.

In conclusion, four ways in which to develop nursing knowledge for the practice of family therapy are explored in this text. There are many other ways this knowledge may be developed, but these four ways are seen as most promising. It is hoped that these exciting theory development efforts will continue and that nurses who practice family therapy will continue to explore these and other theory development methods, so that the knowledge which underlies the societal mandate of nursing may be more fully explicated.

FOUR NURSING APPROACHES TO FAMILY THERAPY

- **Approach One:** Deductive derivation of family therapy approach from a nursing model.
- **Approach Two:** Use of a nursing model to deductively reformulate an existing family therapy theory.
- **Approach Three:** Use of an inductively derived nursing approach to reformulate an existing family therapy theory.
- **Approach Four:** Inductive development of a nursing approach to family therapy.

REFERENCES

Andersen, M. (1982). Personalized nursing: A unique approach to drug dependent women. *Journal of Emergency Nursing, 8*(5), 225–231.

Butler, R., & Lewis, M. (1982). *Aging and mental health: Positive psychosocial and biomedical approaches* (3rd ed.). St. Louis: C.V. Mosby.

Clements, I., & Roberts, F. (1983). *Family health: A theoretical approach to nursing care.* New York: Wiley.

Donaldson, S., & Crowley, D. (1978). The discipline of nursing. *Nursing Outlook, 26,* 113–120.

Ellis, R. (1968). Characteristics of significant theories. *Nursing Research, 17,* 217–222.

Fawcett, J. (1978). The "what" of theory development. In *Theory development: What, why, and how.* New York: National League for Nursing, 17–33.

Fawcett, J. (1983). Hallmarks of success in nursing theory development. In P. Chinn, (Ed.), *Advances in nursing theory development.* Rockville, Md.: Aspen Systems, 3–17.

Johnson, D. (1974). Development of theory: A requisite for nursing as a primary health profession. *Nursing Research, 23,* 372–377.

Kaplan, A. (1963). *The conduct of inquiry.* New York: Harper & Row.

Maslow, A. (1966). *The psychology of science.* South Bend, Ind.: Gateway Editions.

Meleis, A. (1985). *Theoretical nursing: Development and progress.* Philadelphia: J. B. Lippincott.

Popper, K. (1968). *The logic of scientific discovery.* New York: Harper & Row.

Rogers, M. (1970). *An introduction to the theoretical basis for nursing.* Philadelphia: F. A. Davis.

Rogers, M. (1980). Nursing: A science of unitary man. In J. Riehl & C. Roy (Eds.), *Conceptual models for nursing practice* (2nd ed.). New York: Appleton-Century-Crofts.

Schwab, J. (1964). Structure of the disciplines: Meanings and significances. In G. Ford (Ed.), *The structure of knowledge and the curriculum.* Chicago: Rand McNally.

Stevens, B. (1979). *Nursing theory.* Boston: Little, Brown.

Walker, L., & Avant, K. (1983). *Strategies for theory construction in nursing.* Norwalk, Conn.: Appleton-Century-Crofts.

Whall, A. (1980). Congruence between existing theories of family functioning and nursing theories. *Advances in Nursing Science, 3,* 59–67.

Whall, A. (1982). Family system theory: Relationship to nursing conceptual models. In J. Fitzpatrick, A. Whall, R. Johnston, & J. Floyd, (Eds.), *Nursing models and their psychiatric mental health applications.* Bowie, Md.: Brady.

Whall, A. (1985). Clinical research in an academic health center. In *Faculty Practice in Action.* Kansas City, Mo.: American Academy of Nursing.

— APPROACH ONE

Deductive Derivation of Family Therapy Approach From a Nursing Model

2

Approaching Family Intervention through Rogers' Conceptual Model

Ruth L. Johnston

Most of the nursing models or conceptual frameworks which nurses use to derive theories and testable hypotheses to guide research and practice are described as systems approaches. Generally these models address the concepts of person, environment, health, and nursing. In addressing nursing, the activities and process are elaborated in varying degrees to develop the foundations for nursing intervention as well as health promotional activities believed to be an essential part of nursing. Until recently, none of these models addressed directly the issue of family as a unit of study.

The family as an important unit of study for nursing has been emerging historically since the writings of Nightingale (Whall, 1983). Yet the relevance of family to nursing conceptual frameworks has remained largely implicit. Clements and Roberts (1983) review models in terms of their application to families. Their purpose, however, was more to describe family health rather than family therapy approaches. The purpose of this chapter is to describe general ways in which an approach to families in family therapy might be developed through the use of a conceptual framework, specifically that of Rogers.

FOUR WAYS OF VIEWING THE FAMILY

First, four ways of conceptualizing the family are described. Then Rogers' conceptualization of the family system is presented, and the possible compatibility of the four conceptualizations with Rogers' conceptualization is explored. Two existing approaches to families that are based upon

Rogers are reviewed, and changes are made in one approach so as to present an updated guideline for family intervention.

Historically, at least four ways of viewing families have been noted. First, the family may be perceived as the environment of a single individual, a view most prevalent in nursing today. Second, the family interaction between individual family members might be highlighted and the family thus perceived as a group of interacting dyads, triads, etc. Third, the family may be perceived as a single unit or one group, which thinks, feels, and acts in given ways. Fourth, the family may be perceived as a unit which interacts and transacts with its exterior environment (Howells, 1978; Whall, 1981).

These particular views of family may be identified in several existing nursing models. The last two views, at first examination, may seem compatible with the unitary approach of Rogers, however there are discrepancies between these views and the Rogers model. Both the first approach wherein the family is the environment for the individual, and the second approach which focuses upon the interaction of subunits can be useful to the practitioner, but will not be useful in understanding the family as a unit. The third and fourth approaches conceive of the family as a unit, not as interrelated parts, and identify that the family unit acts in ways different from the parts or the action of individual family members. These four ways of viewing the family are roughly similar to those identified by Gillis (1983), except that the last component (i.e., the family as a group interacting with the external environment) is less explicit in Gillis. Rogers views the family as a unit or field which is integral with its environmental field. She differs from other descriptions in the identification of four-dimensionality, rather than describing a three-dimensional family system (Rogers, 1984).

Rogers (1983a) presented a discussion that is helpful in understanding her view of family. She stated that nursing is a sharing of knowledge and skills rather than something one does for, or to, someone else. In addition, "the science of unitary man is a positive developmental approach" (p. 391), and the science of unitary human beings may "differ notably from practices directed toward treating parts . . . or the sum of parts" (p. 390). In discussing a universe of open systems, Rogers indicated that human and environmental fields "flow through one another without interruption" (Rogers, 1983b, p. 222). Thus, in terms of family, no one person would be perceived to have a problem; rather, the entire family and its environment would be defined as client. There is often a linear and causal nature implied in other unitary views of the family which are subtle but nonetheless are inconsistent with Rogers. The unitary nature of the family and the family–environment relationship are described by Rogers as human and environmental fields that "flow through one another without interruption" (Rogers, 1983b, p. 222). In this view of family–environment as energy fields, Rogers eliminates causality and linear relationships from consideration when one approaches family therapy.

An Overview of Rogers' Model

Implications for the Family. In terms of Rogers' principles, the human and environmental fields are identified by wave patterns, and the nature and direction of human and environmental change are continuously innovative with non-repeating rhythmicities characterizing human and environmental fields (Rogers, 1983b). In the view of Rogers, the human and environmental fields change mutually and continuously in a non-causal fashion.

Rogers identified that her model is as applicable to families as it is to individual human beings (Rogers, 1983b). In her view, the family is an irreducible energy field, identified by pattern, and this pattern cannot be identified from the knowledge of individual family members. Also in her view, the family has the capacity to participate knowingly in changes manifesting the family and environmental fields. This self-participation is a creative process and can be directed in terms of family-selected goals (Rogers, 1983b). This optimistic non-manipulative view is summarized in terms of nursing intervention as a creative endeavor in which diversity as well as family knowledge and participation are valued (Rogers, 1983b). Rogers' conceptualization mandates a realistic approach in terms of intervention that would not focus on individual members but rather on the family as an irreducible whole.

The following assumptions of Rogers have been reframed to address families (Rogers, 1970; 1983a,b,c; 1984). This modification is intended to make the conceptual framework more explicit in terms of an understanding of the family system as the unit of care for nursing.

1. The family is a unified whole possessing its own integrity and manifesting characteristics that are different from the sum of the characteristics of the persons who comprise it. The family is a different system and is itself an irreducible field. Viewed as a fundamental unit, the "family" cannot be understood by summing the "parts" or knowledge of the persons who comprise it.
2. Family field and environmental field are in continuous mutual process.
3. The life process of the family evolves irreversibly and innovatively in nonlinear, nonrepeating rhythmicities.
4. Pattern identifies family field; it is the distinguishing characteristic. The nature of the pattern changes continuously and creatively; it is perceived as a single wave.
5. Even as the person is characterized by the capacity for abstraction and imagery, language and thought, sensation and emotion, so too is the family as a whole capable of coherence which is more than and different from that of its members.

Family health in Rogers' approach is not well defined. She has spoken of health as a "value judgment," which does not particularly clarify the concept. Rogers views the term *health* as ambiguous as well as value laden.

Values are continuously changing. *Health* must be recognized, therefore, as a term which in Rogers' view lacks specificity. A synchrony of various patterns between individuals and their family could be interpreted as compatible interpretation of family health with the Rogers' model. A closer view of this interpretation of health, however, demonstrates that it is not a unitary approach and, because *health* lacks specificity in Rogers' view, it cannot be concisely defined (Rogers, 1984).

Health and family health are therefore not defined specifically but are seen as manifestations of family and environmental fields. Health values are manifestations of family and environmental fields. Rogers insists on working with the family, who participate knowingly. Goals are developed with the family, recognizing both family and societal values. Situations such as child abuse are considered in Rogers' view as manifestations of family field/environmental field mutual processes and would be explored as such. A nurse working with a family with child abuse would need to assist the family to participate knowingly in discussions so as to increase their understanding. Selection of patterns for modification and exploration of alternative strategies are key areas upon which the nurse therapist would focus.

Rogers describes nursing as a learned profession, comprising both a science and an art. The science of nursing is the science of unitary persons and unitary families. The art of nursing is the imaginative and creative use of the science of nursing (Rogers, 1983a,b,c; 1984). Families are seen as participating knowingly and probabalistically in the process of change and with the capacity to change.

The assumptions and principles of Rogers' conceptual model give direction for the practice of family therapy by indicating general goals. In Rogers' view, the family is an irreducible, four-dimensional negentropic energy field; family energy fields and their respective environments are in continuous mutual process; "assisting the family in patterning the human field commensurate with improving health is a central goal for nurses" (Rogers, 1983a, p. 390).

Following the view outlined by Rogers, a major step in the nursing care of a family is assessment of the whole. Rogers does not elaborate upon this assessment, but her principles may guide this approach. In order to illuminate Rogers' approach, other approaches by nurse family therapists are discussed to demonstrate differences.

The assessment procedure outlined by Smoyak (1978) offers one view of the family system which is also helpful in understanding the family as a whole. The development of a family genogram and the identification of family rules of organization are examples of Smoyak's approach. The genogram offers an initial step toward intervention in Smoyak's approach. The genogram is discussed as an organized, systematized method for obtaining data about a whole family system for the purpose of identifying patterns of response. Rules of organization, or patterns of interactions, are those patterns which have evolved in a family and which determine who is allowed to do what to whom and with what consequences. This pattern of patterns is seen as being firmly in place, although often without being recognized by the family itself. Smoyak indicates that one should seek evidence of similar rules in the families of origin of the spouses, where recurring patterns can be anticipated (Smoyak, 1978).

At first reading, this approach may seem compatible with the Rogers view. Both are systems approaches; both view the family as a whole, and both discuss patterns. The differences, however, are important. Patterns of family response, as indicated by Smoyak, do not relate to patterns in Rogers' rhythmic sense. Rather, they are recurrences of ways of responding. As the term *response*, in Rogers' view, implies causality, the two approaches are not compatible. Another difference is that, in Rogers' view, "who is allowed to do what to whom" is a focus on parts.

In a Rogers' view, the goal of family therapy is not analysis but rather synthesis. Whereas others speak of "patterns of response," Rogers speaks of pattern in a different context. That is, terms which are used to address analyses in other models are sometimes causal in nature and patterns are seen to *determine* or are a *consequence* (Rogers, 1984). When this is the case, these approaches to family therapy are not compatible with Rogers. The following case presentation is given to demonstrate various ways in which family therapy would and would not be approached from Rogers' perspective.

Case Example

The paternal side of the Murphy family is of Irish descent, the great-grandfather having emmigrated from Ireland to Canada and then to a midwestern industrial city. Characterized by intermarriage with other Irish families, this side of the family consider themselves to be of Irish descent. On the maternal side of the family, a German heritage predominates as several generations of German families have intermarried.

The father, Patrick Murphy, was the only child of Agnes and Timothy Murphy. He is employed as a skilled tradesman. He was married at the age of 25 to Mary Schmitt, also 25 at the time of the marriage. The couple are now in their late 40s and have three children, Maureen, age 17; Joe, age 14; and Tom, age 12. They continue to live in the midst of an industrial city. They consider themselves to be a "normal family" who had little difficulty until Patrick's mother, Agnes, age 74, moved in with them 6 months ago. The move was prompted by the death of Patrick's father from cancer the previous year. Agnes receives less than $2,600 a year as income from Social Security, has no other income and does not own a home. Agnes' home had been sold the previous year to pay the hospital expenses of Timothy. Mary works part-time as a secretary at a local school. The children are all in school and Maureen hopes to attend college next year. The grandmother shares a bedroom with Maureen as the other two bedrooms are occupied respectively by the parents and the two boys.

The presenting problem is the ongoing argument "over everything" between Maureen and her grandmother, resulting in members of the family "taking sides." Patrick sides with his mother, Maureen and Mary side together, and the boys tend to be left out of the arguments. Members of the family would not have come for assistance had not Maureen left home and stayed away for several days on each of two occasions. She complains of no privacy and of Agnes continually criticizing her.

Approach to Family Therapy Consistent with Rogers. General knowledge about a particular cultural group including knowledge of cultural patterns, values, and religious backgrounds does not translate directly into information about this family. Rather, it only serves to alert the nurse to possible patterns, to possible areas of inquiry, and to possible alternative interpretations. Since Rogers' view mandates synthesis rather than analysis, Rogers would consider that examining the needs of each family member would lead to a particulate view of family members, rather than to an appreciation of the integrality of the family–environmental fields.

Assessment would begin by discussing with the family their definition of the family unit and the exploration of the family unit, in terms of such areas as size, nature, and characteristics. Only the family can provide this definition. They alone realize the nature of involvement and the extent of cohesiveness that defines the unit. For some, the nuclear family is the family field, with extended family as a part of the environmental field. For other families, what a therapist might consider extended family, is perceived by the family as themselves integral to their family unit, regardless of numbers involved or the distances of geographic location. Within this system, therefore, the term *family* refers to a range of configurations. For purposes of study, a definition of family field is more or less arbitrary and is defined by the family (Rogers, 1983a).

Nursing has had little experience in defining family units in terms of anything other than individual members. The case history presented above tells us little about the family's perception of the family unit.

Assessment dimensions of the family unit are identified by examining more closely Rogers' building blocks. Four building blocks or concepts have been identified: energy fields, a universe of open systems, pattern, and four-dimensionality (Rogers, 1983b). Energy fields are postulated as the fundamental unit. Energy signifies the dynamic nature of the field. Field is a unifying concept. Two energy fields are identified—the family field and the environmental field (Rogers, 1983b). These are not biologic fields or physical fields or social or psychological fields; they are irreducible yet infinite fields. They are continuously open, integral with each other and with the universe.

A universe of open systems contradicts closed-system concepts such as equilibrium, adaptation, homeostasis and steady-state, and invalidates causality (Rogers, 1983b). These terms would not be used in a Rogerian approach to family therapy. Pattern is the distinguishing characteristic of the family field and is perceived as a single wave, the nature of which changes continuously and innovatively. Four-dimensionality, the least well defined of the concepts, is defined as "a non-linear domain without spatial or temporal attributes. All reality is postulated to be four-dimensional" (Rogers, 1983c, p. 2).

In a non-linear acausal universe of open systems, family fields are viewed as dynamic and in continuous process with the environmental field. The manifestations of this process are another assessment parameter. "Health" and "illness" do not exist as dichotomous entities. They are rather family-defined concepts. Exploration of these concepts of family health–illness and family–field process are helpful as a part of assessment.

A review of the principles guides further the assessment process. The principles of homeodynamics derive from the conceptual system and postulate the nature and direction of change (Rogers, 1983c).

The principle of helicy would posit a constantly evolving family and a constantly evolving environmental field. Although it would be tempting to view the evolving developing rhythms of the family members as dysynchronous, this would be inconsistent with Rogers' model of family. The principle of helicy is manifested in continuous innovative, probabalistic, increasing diversity of family and environmental field patterns. These field patterns are characterized by non-repeating rhythmicities. This principle precludes analytic concepts, such as that of regression of family members. Rather, one looks for and values the increasing diversity of family and environmental field patterns, recognizing similar but increasingly complex patterns. In the case study presented, the family has a "causal view" of the world and of the situation. This leads them to blame-seeking and controlling behaviors that constrict the family view of health. In its failure to recognize and value increasing complexity and diversity, the family may fear change as deviation from accepted norms. This family has identified for themselves weaknesses and conflicts; the nurse will need to identify strengths, indicate the value of diversity, and assist them to understand continuous dynamic change as the expected "norm" of complex systems.

The principle of resonancy concerns a field pattern that is propagated by waves. The continuous change in wave patterns in human and environmental fields is postulated to be from lower to higher frequencies. As the family's life cycle evolves, wave patterns change. In the case history given earlier in this chapter, the family field is presently experiencing an increased diversity of patterns with the entry of Agnes. The system has changed. Past patterns are no longer characteristic of or compatible with the new system.

The principle of integrality postulates mutual process between family and environmental fields. In the case given, the relationship between the developmental process of the family and its environment is important. Although it might be tempting to consider the problem arises from limited sleeping facilities, the need for more space and autonomy for Maureen, and for facilities where Agnes might meet persons of her own age, these assessment–intervention categories are useful in Rogers' view only if the individual is the unit of study. This approach (i.e., examining members needs) is not consistent with Rogers' view of family.

Rather than accept an alien view of the environmental field, the nurse in Rogers' approach identifies a broader range of available resources. In the assessment process, the nurse assists the family to identify problems and goals, and provides opportunities to move from negative to more positive definitions, from a confining to a more open view of the environmental field, and from a generally restrictive to a more accepting view of the changes. Valuing increasing diversity and complexity permits redefinition of the family situation. For this family, the increasing complexity of a new family unit, altered both by the death of Timothy and the introduction of Agnes as live-in family, necessitates considerable redefinition of the family and its goals. The increased diversity is currently expressed by the family through conflicting expectations and hopes and differing views of resources. An evolving coherence is needed for this new system; creative new patterns must be developed. Whall (1981) suggested that the past developmental history of the family is important, because it too is a pattern with relevance for the present situation. Rogers would view the emergence of these new patterns as continuous innovativeness of the process.

In summary, assessment of a family requires a broad view of family field/environmental field. The assessment explores the mutual process of family and environmental field. Rogers views family and environment as irreducible wholes, or systems, "integral with one another and continuously creative in their evolution" (Rogers, 1983b, p. 221). Within this model a family field or system is different from an individual field or system, and the tendency to confuse this issue is seen in the expectation that since parts exist, they must be explained or accounted for within the view of the whole. A study of the parts or particulars increases knowledge of parts, or particulate knowledge; it may be useful to those interested in that level of analysis. It does not relate to knowledge gained from the creative synthesis of facts and ideas and knowledge of the whole.

Within Rogers' conceptual system, the term family refers to a range of configurations. A definition of family field is operational and more or less arbitrary. This arbitrary definition is established through therapist–family exploration and the characteristics of the family are manifestations of the family–environmental process.

Nursing Intervention

Rogers states that "intervention is a creative process in which knowledgeable participation by the family is of central importance" (Rogers, 1984). Diversity is recognized and valued. The nurse is not a part of the family field or of the environmental field within which the process has evolved. The nurse assists the family to define and, if appropriate to their views, redesign the pattern. When families are helped to value diversity and change, perceived "conflict" may be experienced as a challenge to family innovation. Thus, the conflict identified by the family between Agnes and Maureen may be seen as a challenge to the innovation of the family. Open explorations of life-style variations aimed toward family solution of the family-defined conflict would be addressed by the nurse. Valuing of diversity leads to identification of differences as enrichment rather than conflict; the focus thus changes from negative to positive and to innovation rather than blame.

Intervention takes place through shared exploration and support and through an approach that invites the family to present their reasons for seeking assistance. The goal of the nurse is defined in relation to the options and opportunities for family change. Change is facilitated as the family participates in problem definition and pattern modification.

The nurse joins the family and environmental fields. Family and environmental fields are integral with one another; the nurse is integral with the environmental field. The nurse would talk with the Murphy family as a whole, visit the home, and probably hold sessions in the home. The family–environmental field process is more evident within the home and the home is a more natural setting than unfamiliar surroundings. Discussions with the Murphy family would explore any cultural differences as diversity, not deviance. Openness in terms of the discussion of conflicting norms might be a place to begin this discussion with the Murphys. Focus upon positive aspects of both Irish and German heritage, and prizing areas where views are different, might go a long way to begin to assist the Murphy family to change the situation. Diversity in this view is to be anticipated and valued. If diversity is defined as deviance of members, however, change may also be seen as problematic.

Intervention would be discussed by the family, assisted by the nurse. The family sense of the family–environmental system would evolve as family and nurse creatively explore options. The expectations and feelings of the family in terms of the sleeping arrangements are viewed as important. Exploring "reasons" why Maureen found it necessary to leave home would be related to an analytic approach; innovative exploration of options for the whole family is indicated in Rogers' synthesis model, not a focus upon individual motives. The family rules as to who has input into decisions are also less important. Any change in sleeping arrangements would be viewed as a manifestation of family field–environment field process, not in terms of rules and rights. Community resources are also explored by the nurse and family in seeking opportunities for innovation. The family is helped to recognize the evolving diversity of family–environment field process. Family-identified solutions might involve a variety of activities, such as senior groups, boys groups, and other options not available to a family viewing conflict as an insurmountable obstacle. Along with increasing awareness regarding "living space," other innovations could be explored. Is there a room in the basement or attic that the boys could design as a special bunk room for their hobbies and in which they could also sleep? Would this permit Agnes and Maureen to have their own rooms? The exploration would continue until the family is satisfied with the proposed change in pattern.

From a Rogerian perspective, however, family-environment field assessment and intervention through synthesis is more than a single change. The arguments and taking sides which were a focus of the family become less significant as the family explores new options. Rather than making interpretations about what underlying "pathology" is present, the nurse–therapist asks the family to view the arguments as evidence of system diversity, indicating the potential for new patterns which enhance the meeting of family-identified needs. The family is encouraged to identify options and potentials, seeking change as a means of enhancement of the quality of life, rather than fearing change as a threat.

In summary, the family implications identified by Rogers (1983b) are: that the proposed paradigm is as applicable to families as it is to individual human beings; that the family is an energy field, identified by field pattern; and that this field pattern cannot be identified from knowledge of the patterns of individual family members. Also in her view and the view of this author, definition of family is arbitrary, in the sense that the family selects the unit or system for study. A nursing approach to the family derived from Rogers would posit "knowledgeable participation of the family which would lead to changes in the family–environmental field process. This is a creative process and is enhanced by positive attitudes toward change" (Rogers, 1983b). Rogers' approach to family intervention is optimistic and non-manipulative; the approach is a creative endeavor in which diversity is valued as well as family knowledge and participation (Rogers, 1983b).

This Rogerian approach to family therapy assumes that the family is rational and not primarily driven by unconscious motives and desires. The approach also assumes that through shared planning, families may make decisions regarding which, if any, patterns may be modified.

These suggested approaches need to be examined in terms of both the process of therapy and the outcomes of therapy. In addressing this examination new methods of evaluation must be derived for this conceptual system. Such questions as: What are possible negative effects? What ethical questions are involved? and, Is this approach effective? must therefore be asked within the context of this world view. In comparison of this approach with others, i.e., Is this approach as effective, more effective, or less effective? one encounters the problems of causal methodology. That is, causal views of therapy changes are not compatible with Rogers' view. In short, an approach to families may be derived from

Rogers' conceptual model and questions as to the outcomes of this approach need to be explored within this paradigm.

Evaluating Intervention. The nurse might evaluate nursing intervention in terms of the options and potentials identified by the family in making decisions. The question might be asked: Are the new patterns more clearly family decisions rather than decisions by members of the family? Other questions to be asked might be: To what extent did the nurse assist the family to develop criteria for evaluating change? Was the nurse able to focus on facilitating family participation, or was the attempt predominantly one of superimposing preestablished solutions on the family?

Earlier in this chapter the way in which child abuse would be viewed within this conceptual model was discussed. Because the model is an optimistic one and clearly recognizes the role of the family in the decision-making process, the question might be raised, What does the nurse within this model do, if in fact a sexually abusing family indicates that they have no desire to change patterns? Perhaps a vignette will help to illustrate an approach within this conceptual framework:

> The Greene family ask for assistance. They have been referred by the school system for assistance in dealing with the threat that their youngest child, Michael, might be removed from the family because of child abuse. The family generally view this threat as an invasive one on the part of people who "have no right to interfere in how we live and take care of our own. . .".

This family enters the therapeutic situation with a defensive posture—expecting to have to ward off the demands and power of a hostile environment. They have little understanding of the mutual process of family field/environmental field their family patterns reflect. The nurse–therapist in this situation will need considerable skill in non-manipulative, non-threatening approach, in order to engage this family in a shared exploration and a mutual planning for pattern change. The nurse–therapist does not condemn or condone the behaviors but rather explores the present situation as it relates to the self-defined family goals: to keep the family together, and to keep others from forcing change upon them. The societal values and the behavior of social agencies can be predicted. Probable outcomes can be predicted if the family continues to exhibit the current behaviors. The family goals are in conflict; that is, continuation of the abuse will interfere with keeping the family together and will increase the likelihood of additional interference from social agencies. By exploring with this family their view of childrearing patterns, their affective rhythms, and by offering some possible options for altering the present patterns, the nurse–therapist can function in a facilitative, non-manipulative way, helping the family to select the best of available options. Rogers emphasizes that clients have the right to be truly apprised, so that whatever decisions are made are informed ones.

A process of nursing intervention has been presented as it relates to a case presentation, and a limited vignette of a pattern of child abuse. Further discussion of interventions and how they can be derived from this model are needed. This conceptual model was developed emphasizing nursing as a noun and focusing primarily on knowledge development, which is identified by Rogers as the science of nursing. The most common criticism of this conceptual model is in relation to its degree of abstraction and thus limited usefulness. Rogers has, at times, been clearer about what is incompatible with the model, than in presenting guidelines for use of the model. For these reasons, nursing intervention will continue to be explored in case examples, using both Rogers' own work and the efforts of others to implement and extend her conceptual system.

Rogers indicates that family field is a four-dimensional energy field in continuous mutual process with the environmental field, and coextensive with the universe. Boundaries are non-existent, except as arbitrarily placed for purposes of study. She indicates that these perceived boundaries fluctuate such that "... at times the family field may extend further into the environment, and at other times retreat in the direction of a visible core. The nature and intensity of these fluctuating boundaries varies both between families and for given families at different points in time" (Rogers, 1970, p. 90). Family field, then, is both self-defined and fluctuating. Both family field and environmental field boundaries may be perceived to fluctuate. Change in the family field evolves mutually with change in the environmental field. The nurse–therapist enters the perceived environmental field and is thus in a position to facilitate changes in behavior which are manifestations of the family field/environmental field interactive process.

Rogers emphasizes the need for individualized care. With the family, this requires that the nurse see each family as a unique entity; determine the range of behaviors which are "normal" for the family; and prize diversity. Rogers indicates that nursing aims to assist families in achieving maximum health potential. As was indicated previously, "health" is not clearly defined. The term health is seen by Rogers as value laden, individually defined, and socially determined. She is clear that nursing exists to serve people, and that its direct and overriding responsibility is to society (Rogers, 1970). The mutual setting of health goals by the nurse and the family must be framed within the context of the social values within which they are functioning.

Rogers indicates that nursing intervention is always novel because it is designed to meet the needs of the unique human (individual or family) field, in continuous process with its unique environmental field. She states that judicious and wise identification of inventive measures are consonant with the purposes to be achieved in any given situation and that intervention requires the imaginative pulling together of nursing knowledges in new ways according to the particular needs of the individual or group (Rogers, 1970). Helping families to help themselves is a significant facet of nursing practice, and assisting the family in patterning of the family field is commensurate with improving health (Rogers, 1983a).

The Nursing Process and Family Interaction

Fawcett (1984) gives direction and structure to the nursing process within Rogers' conceptual model. She discusses assessment, diagnosis, goal setting, intervention, and evaluation as the elements of the process identified by Rogers in her course materials. Fawcett lists as the areas of assessment: "the simultaneous states of the individual and the environment; the total pattern of events at any given point in space–time; and the rhythms of the life process" (1984, p. 223). She adds as supplemental data, the various disease entities and the subsystem pathology. In the previous discussion of assessment, the family as a unitary whole was the focus, even though some concerns for subsystems (individuals) were expressed. As Fawcett points out, when assessing the individual, disease entities and subsystem pathology are of concern. So too, in family therapy, the nurse must be concerned with the perception by the family of pathology in the subsystems. To focus on pathology separately, however, leads to a distorted view of the whole, but this is not to suggest ignoring its existence when the family believes this is important, or because we do not yet have the vocabulary or the tools to measure these concerns holistically.

Supplementary data concerning the family unit which are particulate in nature may be gathered when the family believes these data are important, so long as they are understood as manifestations of the family field/environmental field relationship. According to Fawcett (1984), in a Rogerian approach when arriving at a nursing diagnosis, the therapist "seeks to identify sequential, cross-sectional patterning in the life process" (1984, p. 223). For example, the Murphy family discussed in the case example was experiencing increasing intensity. The family pattern of blame-seeking led to a constricted view of options, a negative valuing of diversity, and the affective experience of fragmentation rather than coherence.

Goal setting, as elaborated by Fawcett, includes "preservation and enhancement of meaningful life, and meaningful transition from life to death" (1984, p. 223). It is based on consideration of the family as well as society, and the future of man. Goal setting includes the notion of the probabalistic nature of change in man–environment interactions and requires the determination of present and future goals.

Intervention as discussed by Fawcett (1984, p. 223) is: 1) directed toward identification of differences and assisting people to develop patterns of living that are not conflicting with environmental changes; 2) promotion of symphonic interaction between man and environment by identifying field rhythmicities, assisting repatterning for more effective fulfillment of life's capabilities, including humanness, creativeness, capacity as a sentient being, and the symphonic potential of structure and function; 3) strengthening "coherence and integrity of the human field"; and 4) using methods based on "probability of goal achievement." Evaluation can include the need to evaluate the data for the components of the nursing process and to evaluate interventions on the basis of revision of forthcoming or new data.

Interpretations of Family within Rogers' Model

Fawcett's Approach. Fawcett (1975) presented the conceptual view of family as a living open system of coexistensive four-dimensional energy fields. "These energy fields are identified as individuals differentiated from one another by the visible configurations of the fields" (p. 113). She further elaborated the family system as existing as a separate entity similar to the existance of individuals.

Fawcett's conceptual approach to the family is based upon the Rogerian principles of homeodynamics; helicy, synchrony, and resonancy, which she uses to describe the family system. Fawcett (1975) discusses the family and the husband–wife dyad, expanding as children are added to the family. The principle of helicy is defined as the function of continuous innovative change growing out of the mutual interaction of man and environment. For family, helicy is viewed as the family evolving through space–time continuum and organized by specific rhythms. Synchrony is viewed as change in the family system and its environment at a given moment (Fawcett, 1975).

Resonancy is defined by Fawcett as the pattern of energy fields that are the family system and the environment. She continues by stating that wave form characterizes both fields (Fawcett, 1975). Fawcett further elaborated these principles as they related to family, substituting complementarity for synchrony, as Rogers had in her conceptual model (Fawcett, 1979).

For Fawcett (1975), the Rogers' model provides a view of family as an interacting whole and fosters a comprehensive view of family life and consequently fosters more comprehensive intervention. As Rogers' conceptualization for guiding nursing research, she cautions that "measurement devices present special problems, and it seems probable that artificial dichotomies will have to be employed until four-dimensional measurement tools are developed" (p. 116). In her research, Fawcett (1977, 1978) continues to address some of these concerns.

Whall's Assessment of Families. Further development of the conceptualization of family within Rogers' conceptual model is offered by Whall (1981). Building upon Fawcett's work, Whall presents an assessment model for families. In her elaboration of the principles of homeodynamics as explicated for families by Fawcett, Whall discusses that the principle of helicy is illustrated by the family evolving unidirectionally with the rhythms of birth, growth to adulthood, and death. "No one ever gets younger" (Whall, 1981, p. 31). Complementarity, or the interaction of family field and environmental field, is mutual and simultaneous; each is affected by the evolving of the other. Resonancy is defined as "change in pattern and organization which is propagated by waves" (p. 31). This is exemplified by the wave pattern in the extended family system as new units are formed, children are born, grow into adulthood, and give birth to more children. The increasing complexity of the principle of helicy is also evident in the evolving patterns.

Following Fawcett's (1975) discussion of the family as an open system composed of interrelated parts or subsystems which are individual members, Whall (1981) assesses family subsystems. She offers as rationale that "if one understands that the whole can never in any additive fashion equal the sum of the parts, and if one understands that the parts are essentially 'boundaryless,' then it is possible to consider individual family members in the assessment" (Whall, 1981, p. 32). She emphasizes that the perspective of this assessment be focused upon the whole family system; that identification of subsystem characteristics is for the purpose of identification of the configuration of the whole. Whall believes that this approach can lead to identification of the patterns of the whole; and is a necessary approach because the nurse cannot observe the four-dimensional energy field that is the family (Whall, 1981, p. 32). From the assessment of the parts the process proceeds to focus on the unique characteristics of the whole, or the way in which the whole family acts as a unit.

In this approach, the assessment moves to the environmental field and the family field/environmental field interaction. Whall's assessment guideline for families is further elaborated to include the areas of assessment with each category indicated. A basic assumption is made that each person and family is characterized by rhythmic developmental sequences which are patterning and repatterning in mutual simultaneous interaction with the environment. These dimensions are essentially boundaryless and thus an overlap will appear to occur.

In considering the individual subsystems, Whall (1981) first looks at developmental considerations. More specifically, she examines the past developmental history of parents and children including the parents' physical and emotional health at the time of establishing the family unit. Additional developmental landmarks such as age, specific tasks, and physical growth for each person are noted. Psychosexual development of each member is considered; a history of life traumas and present level of functioning in developmental tasks are noted for each member.

Biological considerations include the general state of health of each member, past and present difficulties and care; past and present physical level of functioning as well as genetic factors affecting the level of functioning. Psychological considerations include the general state of emotional health and psychological growth, past and present problems, and general level of functioning with regard to cognitive and affective elements. Assessment of social dimensions includes class and cultural factors, with attention to support systems, general social development of children and adults, and finally, the nurse as an individual and what she/he brings to the situation such as values, biases, development, etc.

The second major category, interactional patterns, includes assessment of executive and sibling relationships, i.e., clear versus breached generational levels; negotiation patterns and levels; triadic and dyadic relationships including positive and negative relationships, and the cyclic nature of behavioral sequencing. Assessment of interaction patterns includes communication patterns, looking for clarity versus distortions such as double messages, and identification of the usual channels and modes of communication. Role relationships include role reciprocity or role confusion and inconsistency; complementarity or symmetrical patterns, and ways in which intimacy is expressed. Attachment patterns may include commitment and detachment levels, individuation and enmeshment levels, mutuality and isolation levels, and explicit and implicit expectations.

Unique characteristics of the whole are assessed as Whall suggests looking first at the family group psyche, including relative stability or disorganization, and the capacity for change such as relative flexibility or rigidity. Belief systems of the family include values, myths (including distortion, such as sham and pseudomutuality), and rules regarding expression of beliefs. Group dynamic characteristics, such as power structure, leadership, and problem-solving ability, cohesiveness and reference groups, and "boundary" characteristics—who is allowed "in" and who is "out," are also assessed. Family development needs including both maturational and situational requirements are assessed. Family actions may be categorized as open, random, or more rigid life-styles. Economic factors are an important assessment area. These may include: distribution of income, income as related to needs, and style of disbursement.

The fourth major category, that of family field/environmental field interaction or environmental interface synchrony, looks at family developmental needs as they relate to community resources; family values compared to community values and beliefs; community demands upon the family, and the effect of the family upon the community.

This assessment guide is intended to be reflective of the main concepts of Rogers' model. That Fawcett agrees with this approach is implicit in her statement that "Whall constructed a logically congruent conceptual–theoretical system of nursing knowledge from Rogers' conceptual model, Fawcett's extension of Rogers' model to the family system and theories of family functioning" (Fawcett, 1984, p. 232).

Newman (1979) offers the following questions to guide as a critique of a holistic view: Does the assessment reflect pattern and organization specific to the individual family? Does the pattern and organization presented reflect rhythmicity and unidirectionality? Does it include the essential elements of identification of sequential, cross-sectional patterning in the life process? Specific assessment of individuals, in the assessment of biological, psychological, and social dimensions, would, however, be viewed by Rogers as a particulate approach.

Both Whall and Fawcett have moved the process forward through their efforts to derive approaches from Rogers' very abstract model, and both have done so prior to some of the more recent clarification of model concepts and relationships. It is clear that both are attempting to identify a process that will make family system assessment possible. It is equally clear that both bring to this process the view of an experienced practitioner and theorist.

The Whall Model Revisited. To reformulate Whall's approach it is important to begin with an assessment of the unitary family. To begin with an assessment of individuals reinforces the older perspective of particulate man. Some way of assessing aspects of the whole is offered (see Fig. 2–1). The modification presented in Figure 2–1 has the limitation of presenting the particulate within the whole. A more accurate representation would

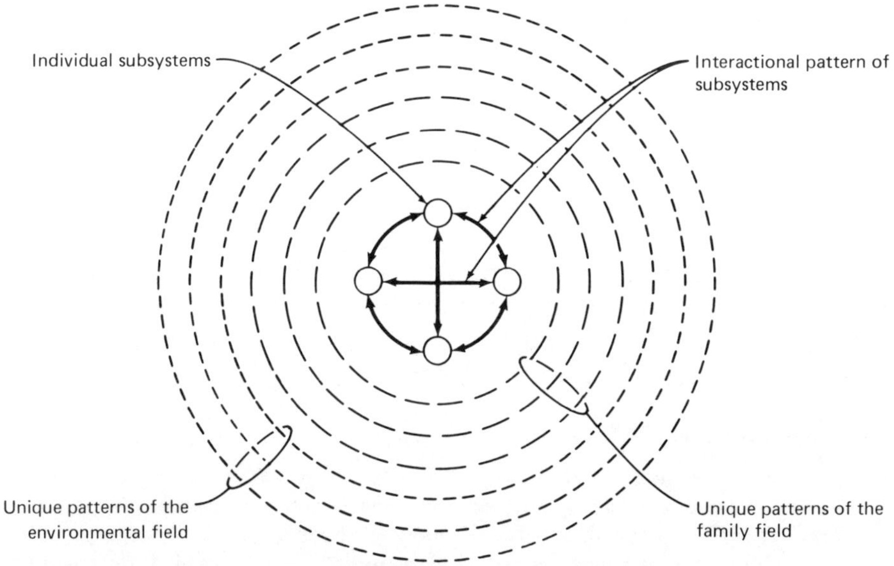

Figure 2–1. Adaptation of a nursing model for family assessment. **Note:** In a more accurate representation of this figure, when the individual subsystems could be seen, the whole would be invisible, and when the whole could be seen, the subsystems would be invisible. *(From Whall A. L. (1981). Journal of Psychiatric Nursing and Mental Health Services,* 19, *32.)*

TABLE 2-1. AN ASSESSMENT GUIDELINE FOR WORK WITH FAMILIES

The assumption is made that the family is characterized by rhythmic developmental sequences which are in mutual process with the environmental field. Family field and environmental fields are four-dimensional energy fields in continuous interaction, integral with each other, and coextensive with the universe. Family field and environmental fields are essentially boundaryless, are unique.

The family unit:

- Definition of family, by the family:
  - Perceived boundary characteristics—who is allowed "in" and who is "out"
  - Problem-solving patterns; style
  - Typological actions (centripetal and/or centrifugal)
  - Capacity to validate reality
  - Coherence; the "sense" of family
- Family organization identified by the family:
  - Relative stability and/or disorganization
  - Capacity for change
  - Family power structure
  - Leadership, problem-solving abilities
  - Cohesiveness; reference groups
- Belief systems identified by the family:
  - Patterns of valuing
  - Patterns of sharing/communicating beliefs
- Family developmental needs identified by the family:
  - Maturational requirements
  - Situational requirements
- Economic factors identified by the family:
  - Patterns of income distribution
  - Income as related to values/needs
  - Patterns/style of disbursement

---

show that when individual subsystems are visible, the whole can not be seen, and when the whole is visible the parts cannot be seen.

Following this approach, modification of Whall's assessment guideline for work with families is presented. To offer further clarification regarding the way in which supplemental data indicated in Table 2–1 might be used in a Rogerian approach, the following vignette is presented:

Case Example

John and Sue Lee, a couple in their mid 40s, have two teenage children. Recently, Sue was diagnosed as having breast cancer. She was successfully treated with a simple mastectomy followed by reconstructive surgery. In the family assessment there were no obvious indications that this family was experiencing cancer. Yet, in discussions, Sue offered the information that she has experienced cancer of the breast. The recency of the event had left the family hesitant to initiate this discussion. When the therapist facilitated this exploration, family patterns were identified, goals for repatterning were formulated, and additional resources were made available to the family.

- Family field/environmental field complementarity, identified by the family:
  - Developmental needs of family—community resources
  - Family patterns of valuing—community patterns of valuing
  - Family expectations of community—community expectations
  - Support systems
- Supplemental data[a] identified by the family:
  - Health assessment of subsystems (individual members) to be sure family assessment is complete
  - Developmental/situational/maturational factors obvious for individuals, not yet clear as family system patterns
  - Executive and sibling system interactions
    - Clear—breached generational levels
    - Patterns of negotiation
  - Triadic and dyadic relationships
    - Positive and negative vectors in relationships
    - Patterns of negotiation
- Communication patterns
  - Role relationships
    - Role reciprocity and/or role confusion and inconsistency
    - Complementarity and/or symmetrical patterns
    - Patterns of expression of intimacy
  - Attachment patterns
    - Commitment and detachment levels
    - Individuation and/or enmeshment patterns
    - Patterns of mutuality and/or isolation
    - Implicit and explicit expectations

[a]Supplemental data, gathered in a particulate way, are recognized as a contradiction to Rogers' model. This assessment is offered as a transitional step in evolving unitary family assessment. These data should guide the framing of questions to elicit family system data which were previously overlooked and became apparent only in a particulate assessment.

(Modified from Whall, A. L. (1981). Journal of Psychiatric Nursing and Mental Health Services, 19, *33–34.)*

Although it is necessary to learn to think in terms of families experiencing cancer, just as we are beginning to accept a "pregnant family," this family information would not have become available had not the mother been seen separately. Particulate information can be transformed, or "reformulated" to become holistic in nature if it is used to guide an approach to overall family patterns. Environmental data may also come to the therapist in a particulate way. The need to continue the assessment as an ongoing process leading to the identification of family patterns and the mutual family field/environmental field process as it evolves is of paramount importance. In no way does this recommend the treatment of the family as other than an irreducible open system.

SUMMARY

An approach to family therapy has been presented which is derived from Fawcett and Whall and which is consistent with Rogers' model. Initially, various ways of viewing the family were discussed as compatible or incompatible with Rogers' model. Rogers' model was reviewed for indications of ways in which family therapy would or would not be approached within the model. Two existing approaches to families which are based upon Rogers' model were reviewed. Case examples were presented throughout. Discussions of the ways in which the four central concepts of nursing are viewed in this derived approach to family therapy are discussed throughout the chapter. It is hoped that these attempts will assist with the development of a family therapy approach consistent with Rogers' model.

RESEARCH

Although little research has been done on Rogers' approach to family, a growing body of research on the model is available. References not cited in this chapter are offered as additional sources of information and understanding of the "state of the art" in investigating this complex model, although not all these sources are research per se.

FOUR CENTRAL COMPONENTS OF NURSING APPROACHES

- **Title of Chapter:** Approaching Family Intervention through Rogers' Conceptual Model
- **Definitions**
- **Family:** A four-dimensional, irreducible energy field; a unified whole possessing its own integrity and manifesting characteristics that are more than and different from the sum of characteristics of the persons who comprise it. Pattern identifies family field; it is the distinguishing characteristic. The nature of the pattern changes continuously and creatively; it is perceived as a single wave.
- **Family Environment:** A four-dimensional energy field in continuous mutual process with family field. Family field and environmental field are integral with each other. Environment field includes all that is external to the family field.
- **Family Health:** Rogers views *health* as an ambiguous as well as value-laden term. Values are continually changing. Family health can be defined with specificity with a given family at a particular time.
- **Therapist's Approach:** Intervention is a creative process in which the knowledgeable participation by the family is of central importance; pattern diversity is recognized and valued, and identified pattern change is experienced as a challenge to innovation.

REFERENCES

Clements, I. W., & Roberts, F. B. (Eds.), (1983). *Family health: A theoretical approach to nursing care.* New York: Wiley.

Fawcett, J. (1975). The family as a living open system: An emerging conceptual framework for nursing. *International Nursing Review, 22,* 113–116.

Fawcett, J. (1977). The relationship between identification and patterns of change in spouses' body images during and after pregnancy. *International Journal of Nursing Studies, 14,* 199–213.

Fawcett, J. (1978). Body image and the pregnant couple. *American Journal of Maternal Child Nursing,* July/August, pp. 227–233.

Fawcett, J. (1979). The family as a living open system. Lecture at Wayne State University, College of Nursing, Detroit, Michigan, May 18, 1979.

Fawcett, J. (1984). *Analysis and evaluation of conceptual models of nursing.* Philadelphia: F. A. Davis.

Gillis, C. (1983). The family as a unit of analysis: Strategies for the nurse researcher. *Advances in Nursing Science, 5,* 50–59.

Howells, J. (1978). Family psychiatry workshop. Presentation to Northwest Hospital Association and Michigan Psychiatric Society, Detroit, Michigan, November, 1978.

Newman, M. (1979) *Theory development in nursing.* Philadelphia: F. A. Davis.

Rogers, M. E. (1970). *An Introduction to the theoretical basis of nursing.* Philadelphia: F. A. Davis.

Rogers, M. E. (1983a). Analysis and application of Rogers' theory of nursing. In I. W. Clements & F. B. Roberts, (Eds.), *Family health: A theoretical approach to nursing care* (pp. 390–391). New York: Wiley.

Rogers, M. E. (1983b). Science of unitary human beings: A paradigm for nursing. In I. W. Clements & F. B. Roberts (Eds.), *Family health: A theoretical approach to nursing care* (pp. 219–228). New York: Wiley.

Rogers, M. E. (1983c). *Science of unitary human beings: A paradigm for nursing.* Unpublished class materials.

Rogers, M. E. (1984). Personal communication, June, 1984.

Smoyak, S. (1978). Family systems: Use of genograms as an assessment tool. In Proceedings of the Twenty-Fifth Annual Conference of Air Force Behavioral Scientists, May, 1978.

Whall, A. L. (1981). Nursing theory and the assessment of families. *Journal of Psychiatric Nursing and Mental Health Services, 19,* 30–36.

Whall, A. L. (1983). The family focus in nursing: A historical perspective. Paper presented at the Nursing Theory Think Tank, Chicago, September, 1983.

Additional References

Blair, C. (1979). Hyperactivity in children: Viewed within the framework of synergistic man. *Nursing Forum, 18,* 293–303.

Boguslawski, M. (1979). The use of therapeutic touch in nursing. *Journal of Continuing Education in Nursing, 10*(4), 9–15.

Engle, V. (1981). Movement and time as correlates of health. Paper presented at ANA Council of Nurse Researchers Annual Meeting. Washington, D. C., September, 1981.

Fitzpatrick, J. J. (1980). Patients' perceptions of time: Current research. *International Nursing Review, 27*, 148–153, 160.

Fitzpatrick, J. J. (1982). The crisis perspective: Relationship to nursing. In J. J. Fitzpatrick, A. L. Whall, R. L. Johnston, & J. A. Floyd, (Eds.), *Nursing models and their psychiatric mental health applications*. Bowie, Md.: Brady.

Fitzpatrick, J. J. Whall, A. L., Johnston, R. L., Floyd, J. A. (Eds.) (1982). *Nursing models and their psychiatric mental health applications*. Bowie, Md.: Brady.

Gill, B. P., & Atwood, J. R. (1981). Reciprocy and helicy used to relate mEGF and wound healing. *Nursing Research, 30*, 68–72.

Heidt, P. (1981). Effect of therapeutic touch on anxiety level of hospitalized patients. *Nursing Research, 30*, 32–37.

Johnston, R. L., Fitzpatrick, J. J., & Donovan, M. J. (1982). Developmental stage: Relationship to temporal dimensions (abstract). *Nursing Research, 31*, 120.

Kreiger, D. (1975). Therapeutic touch: The imprimatur of nursing. *American Journal of Nursing, 75*, 784–787.

Kreiger, D. (1981). *Foundations for holistic health nursing practice: The renaissance nurse*. Philadelphia: J. B. Lippincott.

McDonald, S. (1981). Visible lightwaves and the experience of pain (abstract). Paper presented at ANA Council of Nurse Researchers, Washington, D. C., 1981.

Macrae, J. (1979). Therapeutic touch in practice. *American Journal of Nursing, 79*, 664–665.

Malinski, V. (1980). The relationship between hyperactivity in children and perception of short wave length light: An investigation into the conceptual system proposed by Martha E. Rogers. Ph.D. dissertation, New York University.

Miller, L. A. (1979). An explanation of therapeutic touch using the science of unitary man. *Nursing Forum, 18*, 278–287.

Moore, G. (1982). Perceptual complexity, memory and human duration experience. (abstract) *Nursing Research, 31*, 189.

Quinn, J. (1984). Therapeutic touch as energy exchange: Testing a theory. *Advances in Nursing Science, 6*, 42–49.

Reed, P. G., Fitzpatrick, J. J., Donovan, M. J., & Johnston, R. L. (1982). Suicidal crises: Relationship to the experience of time (abstract). *Nursing Research, 31*, 122.

3

Family Therapy as Derived from King's Conceptual Model

Paula W. Gonot

A basic premise underlying family therapy is that symptoms exhibited by an individual are both a signal and a function of a disturbance in the family system (Peplau, 1975). This perspective of the family as a system and as the focus of therapy is consistent with Imogene M. King's conceptual framework for nursing (1981). By King's own formulation (1983), her model is amenable to developing a theoretical approach to the care of families. The purpose of this chapter is to deduce a theoretical model for family therapy from King's conceptual framework and theory of goal attainment, drawing upon and extending King's formulations (1981, 1983).

THEORETICAL MODEL

King's conceptual framework (1981) is composed of three interacting systems—personal, interpersonal, and social. Individuals are personal systems. When individuals form groups, this formation constitutes interpersonal systems. Groups with common interests and goals create social systems within society (King, 1981). The concepts presented as substantive content for nursing in each of the three interacting systems of the framework are as follows (King, 1981, pp. xi–xii):

Personal	**Interpersonal**	**Social**
Perception	Human interactions	Organization
Self	Communication	Authority
Growth and development	Transactions	Power
Body image	Role	Status
Space	Stress	Decision making
Time		

From a systems perspective, the interpersonal system is the focal system of King's framework. Personal systems, i.e., individuals, are the components or subsystems of interpersonal systems. Social systems designate the various environments or suprasystems in which interpersonal systems are experienced. The concepts identified in both personal and social systems serve to enhance one's understanding of interpersonal systems (Gonot, 1983). This perspective parallels a systems approach to families. Individual members are the subsystems of the focal system of the family. The social systems of the society, such as support networks, schools, religious groups, neighborhoods, and health care agencies, comprise the environmental suprasystem of the family system. To understand the family, one must have knowledge of the individual family members as well as the suprasystem within which the family functions.

Family Unit

Conceptualized within King's model, the family is an interpersonal system, a group of individuals interacting to meet their basic needs. Through communication and perception of the internal and external environment, family members interact purposefully toward transactions, i.e., the attainment of goals. As an open system exhibiting permeable boundaries, the family exchanges matter, energy, and information with the environment for the regulation and control of stressors (King, 1981).

The family is simultaneously a social system exhibiting organization, authority, power, status, and decision making (King, 1983). The family provides the initial process of socialization for the individual, teaching beliefs, attitudes, values, and customs, and establishing rules of behavior and modes of action (King, 1981). King submits that while the structure of the family system will vary from one society and culture to another, "there is some structure in every society" (1983, p. 180). Whether viewing the family as an interpersonal system or a social system, King's formulations are applicable to various family structures—from nuclear to single parent to childless units—regardless of biological and legal relatedness.

King (1983) proposes the conceptualization of family as an interpersonal system in terms of therapy. As the focus of her framework, relatively greater detail is provided the description of concepts within interpersonal systems. The theory of goal attainment that King deduced from the model (1981) is derived primarily from this system. Further, the theory of goal attainment represents, in essence, King's formulations of the nursing process within which the interpersonal system of nurse–client is experienced (Gonot, 1983). In the case of family therapy, the client is the family system.

When describing the interpersonal system of nurse–client in both the conceptual framework and the theory of goal attainment, King attends to each participant in the system. The perception, judgment, action, and reaction of each individual party is taken into account in the process of human interactions (King, 1981). Correspondingly, King's formulation of the family encompasses characteristics of the family members, or subsystems, as well as the family system. These characteristics include King's philosophical assumptions about human beings: individuals are social beings, sentient beings, rational beings, reacting beings, perceiving beings, controlling beings, action-oriented beings, and time-oriented beings (1981). Family members, as individuals comprising the family system, have rights and responsibilities. These formulations and assumptions guide the nurse–therapist in working with families.

Family Health

Health is "a high priority in the hierarchy of values in society," a process of growth and development that is not always smooth or without conflict (King, 1981, pp. 4–5). Extending King's (1981) definition of health from the individual to the family system yields this description of family health: dynamic life experiences which imply continuous adjustment to stressors in the internal and external environment through optimum use of family resources to achieve maximum potential for daily living.

Stressors may emanate from biological, psychological, social, and cultural sources. Health relates to the ways individuals and family systems deal with the stressors of growth and development while functioning within the cultural pattern in which they are born and to which they attempt to conform (King, 1981, 1983).

More concisely, health is the ability to function in social roles (King, 1981). Family members enact a variety of roles internal to the system and within the suprasystem. Familial roles include spouse, lover, parent, sibling, child, confidante, provider, and caretaker. External roles will vary with the position(s) one holds, such as administrator, nurse, faculty, technician, student, volunteer. The degree to which family members are able to function in roles while dealing with stressors reflects the health of the family. Whereas health is viewed as a functional state in the life cycle, illness indicates an interference in the cycle. An interference experienced by one or more family members will have an impact on the health status of the family system.

Environment

The environment is also conceptualized as an open system that exhibits permeable boundaries permitting an exchange of matter, energy, and information with human beings. Satisfaction in the performance of daily living depends upon harmony and balance in each person's environment. The interpersonal system of the family is the immediate social environment of the individual (King, 1981, 1983). The essential variables King identifies in the interaction between nurse and client are also characteristic of the family system. These include the geographical place of the interacting subsystems, the spacial–temporal dimensions, the perceptions, expectations, roles, and communications of the members, the stressors being experienced within the system, and the established family goals (King, 1981).

The external environment is the suprasystem in which the family functions. There are various aspects of the suprasystem including all the personal, interpersonal, and social systems with which the family system interacts. The family's adjustment to its internal environment will affect its relationship with the external environment, and vice versa. Understanding the ways families interact with their environment to maintain health is essential to the nurse–therapist. The environment is not to be viewed as that to which the family must conform. King submits that "the moving forces in nursing are imbedded in the dynamics of society in which the process of change alters the environment" (1981, p. 11).

Role of the Nurse–Therapist

King has delineated the domain of nursing as the "promotion of health, maintenance and restoration of health, care of the sick and injured, and care of the dying" (1981, p. 4). To accomplish this, the nurse develops an interpersonal system with the client family in which the traditional steps of the nursing process are carried out. The nurse examining the data (assessment) in order "to plan, implement, and evaluate nursing care is the function of the professional nurse" (King, 1981, p. 9).

The theory of goal attainment which King deduced from her conceptual model describes the nursing process in the context of an interpersonal system of nurse and client. Within this system, the elements of the human interaction process are experienced. The nurse–therapist and the family members perceive and make mental judgments about one another. Through observation and purposeful communication, the nurse–therapist elicits, interprets, and shares information with the family. As family members share their perceptions and concerns, real or potential problems are identified. The nurse–therapist engages the participation of the family in the determination of goals and the means to achieve them. All subsystems—each family member and the nurse–therapist—must come to mutually agree upon the goals of therapy. For if family health is to be promoted, transactions must occur.

To paraphrase King's statement (1981) of the interrelationships of person, environment, health, and nursing from the perspective of family: the focus of family therapy is the family system interacting with its environment leading to a state of health, which is the ability to function in social roles.

THERAPEUTIC PROCESS

Approaching the Family

Prior to approaching the family system, the nurse–therapist must be aware of the philosophical assumptions and professional values he/she holds about human beings, the therapeutic process, and the practice of nursing. In the section on family health in this chapter, the philosophical assumptions within King's framework about the nature of human beings were presented. King (1981) has also explicated assumptions regarding the nurse–client interaction and nursing practice, some of which are set forth in the ANA *Code for Nurses* (1976) and *Standards for Nursing Practice* (1973). Specific assumptions and values about the nurse–client (family) interaction process are:

- Perceptions of nurse and of client influence the process.
- Goals, needs, and values of nurse and of client influence the process.
- Individuals have a right to knowledge about themselves.
- Individuals have a right to participate in decisions that influence their life, health, and community services.
- Health professionals have a responsibility to share information so that individuals may make informed decisions about their health care.
- Individuals have a right to accept or reject health care.
- Goals of health professionals and goals of recipients of health care may be incongruent (King, 1981, pp. 143–144).

The practice model, as derived from King's formulations, is congruent with these assumptions. The nurse–therapist's interaction with the family system is reflective of the philosophical stance and professional values. When the nurse interacts with the family, factors associated with the professional's role and the rights and responsibilities of clients are presented as the ground rules for their interaction.

Nurses come in contact with families in a variety of settings under a myriad of circumstances, though not all interactions are purposeful or systematic (King, 1983). Nurse–client interactions that have the potential of leading to transactions are those pertinent to the family's health state. Whether concerns or problems initially were recognized by the family member(s) or were brought to their attention by a third party is not determinantal. It is essential, however, that the members either acknowledge their concern(s) or are willing to explore the possibility of real or potential problems. "Perception is a key concept in dealing with families and their health" (King, 1983, p. 181). While it is one of a number of component concepts of the theory of goal attainment guiding the nursing process, King submits that perception is perhaps the most basic determinant of behavior (1981, 1983).

There may be some instances where one or more family members perceive a problem and other member(s) do not. When incongruence in perception persists and some members are unwilling to interact and participate, those seeking therapy may choose to participate without the others. Though the family system as a whole does not benefit as directly, some change may be affected as one or more members establish and attain health-related goals. There may also be cases where individual therapy is warranted for member(s) collateral to family therapy.

Assessment

The theory of goal attainment was deduced primarily from concepts described within the interpersonal system of King's framework (1981). The theory, which embodies the nursing process, provides a useful framework for guiding practice. In assessing the interpersonal system of the family as well as nurse–client (family), the nurse–therapist gathers facts through communication, observations, and measurements about all the concepts in the theory of goal attainment. "Each of the concepts in the theory are interrelated and influence every person's behavior" (King, 1983, p. 183). A problem in any one conceptual area has implications for the entire interaction process. The concepts of the theory of goal attainment are interactions, perception, communication, transaction, role, stress, and growth and development (King, 1981).

Interaction. The process of interaction in the interpersonal system of both the family and nurse–client has been discussed previously in this chapter. The structure and composition of the interacting system are assessed in terms of the number of subsystems and the relationships of the subsystems. Who are the family members and how are they related? Because interpersonal systems are, by definition, the interaction of two or more persons, assessment of the remaining concepts as experienced within the family system is fundamental to understanding the interaction process. The nurse–therapist must keep in mind that, while assessing the system of the family, the therapist is also a subsystem of the interpersonal system of nurse and client. As such, the perceptions and communications of the therapist are significant factors in the assessment process.

Perception. Perception is each person's representation of reality, an awareness of persons, objects, and events. It is subjective, personal, and selective. Perception gives meaning to one's experience and influences one's behavior (King, 1981). The nurse–therapist assesses the perception of each family member as to the concerns or problems each one is experiencing. What does each member perceive to be the reason for seeking therapy? Assessment focuses on members' perceptions of their needs, values, and goals. Are needs being met? What seems to be of value to the individuals and to the family system? Are the goals individual or shared? One person's perception may be affected by what is perceived to be other persons' perceptions. How does each member perceive the perceptions of other members? Are the perceptions congruent? If not, the nurse assesses how family members react to differing perceptions.

Communication. One communicates on the basis of perceptions. Accuracy of perception increases effectiveness of one's actions. The informational component of interactions is communication. "Communication is the structure of significant signs and symbols that bring order and meaning to human interaction" (King, 1981, p. 62). Universal characteristics are that communication is verbal, non-verbal, situational, perceptual, transactional, and irreversible (King, 1981). At times, more important than the actual content of the message is the relationship implied between the interacting persons. The nurse–therapist learns much about how the family members interact by observing the communication patterns. Is the communication clear or ambiguous? Are verbal and non-verbal behaviors consistent or contradictory? When one individual is talking, do the others listen? Is each family member given the opportunity for expression? If communications are not open, clear, and consistent, the interaction process is stifled.

Transaction. Whereas communication is the transfer of information, transaction is the transfer of value between two or more persons. Both kinds of interaction are necessary to promote health. Transaction is "a process of interaction in which human beings communicate with the environment to achieve goals that are valued" (King, 1981, pp. 81–82). The immediate environment of each family member is the family system. If there are problems in perception and communication, the values will not be shared nor goals negotiated.

Role. The concept of role is relevant to each member individually as well as to the family system. Individuals enact familial roles and roles related to positions held in the suprasystem. Because the ability to function in social roles is a reflection of health, assessment in this area is fundamental. Glasser and Glasser (1970) contend that consistency of individual role expectations for oneself and others in the system is a basic requirement for adequate family functioning. Further, roles and expected behaviors should be fairly constant throughout time lest the internal functioning of the family be unsteady. The nurse–therapist assesses whether or not role expectations are consistent within the family. Are members behaving in accord with expectations? Is a change in roles being experienced by one or more individuals—either within the system or in the suprasystem? The degree of satisfaction with roles is also assessed. Role dissatisfaction could manifest itself as dissatisfaction with actual membership in the family.

Stress. An element of stress is essential for human functioning and health (King, 1983). Throughout the lifespan one may be faced with a myriad of stressful events, e.g., bereavement, entering school, illness, pregnancy, unemployment, marriage, career change, bankruptcy, child leaving home, relocation. Inherent in any stressful event or situation is the potential for precipitating a crisis. Crisis is defined as occurring when a person faces an obstacle to important life goals that is, for a time, unsurmountable through customary methods of problem solving (Caplan, 1961). Previous successes in dealing with stressful events increase the likelihood of subsequent successes. The literature suggests that perception of the event, coping mechanisms or resources, and supportive interpersonal relationships are significant variables in determining whether or not a stressful event leads to a crisis (Aguilera & Messick, 1974). Families in therapy may be experiencing a number of stressful events with which they are feeling unable to deal. Too many stressors in the family environment may precipitate a crisis (King, 1983). If just one individual is in a state of crisis, the family system experiences a heightened level of stress. Each member's perception of what is going on in the family is crucial to assessment. Are members attributing their situation to any one family member? Has that individual assumed responsibility for the identified problem? It is important that the nurse–therapist ascertain the degree to which the stressful event has affected individual and system functioning. Has role performance been impaired? Have the activities of daily living been altered? Are members seemingly supportive of one another? Assessment includes an historical perspective on the occurrence of stressful events. How does the family customarily deal with stress? Is there an identifiable pattern of coping? What is similar and dissimilar about the present experience?

Growth and Development. Crises have been categorized into two groups: "the unexpected, accidental, situational crises that are not anticipated; and the expected, developmental, maturational crises that occur as persons grow and develop" (Barrell, 1974, p. 7). Problems in the area of growth and development are most likely to be related to a maturational crisis of one or more family members. Maturational crises occur during periods of great social, physical, and psychological change and often necessitate role transitions (Aguilera & Messick, 1974). Rigid perception is often the source of difficulties in making role changes. If either the individual is unable to picture self in the new role or significant others refuse to see the person in a different role, the state of crisis will not be resolved (Williams, 1971). For as King notes (1981), the manner in which a person grows and develops may be influenced either positively or negatively by other people and objects in the environment. Again, assessment focuses on perception. How is the role transition viewed by the family members? Has the imminence of the maturation been accepted? The notion of role reciprocity raises another question regarding maturational crises—who is in crisis? For example, as the child develops into adulthood, what becomes of the parent role? Exploring what the event means to each family member yields valuable data. Specific interview questions are guided by the developmental stage of the individuals.

The nurse–therapist is cognizant of the interrelatedness of the concepts of the model as applied to the interpersonal system of the family

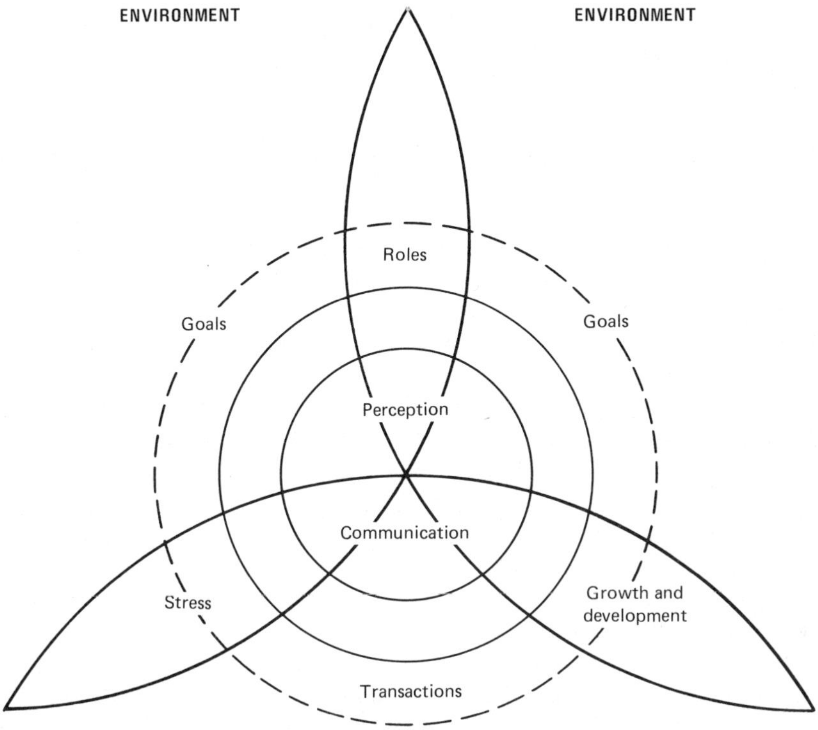

Figure 3-1. Interpersonal system of the family—Assessment components in therapy.

(Fig. 3–1). Throughout the assessment process, observations are made as to the manner in which perceptions and values are communicated and the family members' reactions to information shared.

Nursing Diagnoses

The nurse–therapist synthesizes the assessment data with the knowledge base of the discipline. Diagnoses are derived which emanate from one or more of the conceptual areas of: interaction, perception, communication, transaction, role, stress, and growth and development. The interrelatedness of the concepts is demonstrated in the following examples:

- Situational crisis precipitated by stress of unemployment and subsequent role reversal
- Incongruent perceptions of goals resulting from lack of open communication
- Rigid perception and unwillingness to relinquish role leading to maturational crisis

- Inadequate role performance heightened by stress of relocation and incongruent goals

Intervention and Evaluation

The nurse–therapist's initial intervention is upon introduction to the family system. By interacting with the family members, the nurse forms an interpersonal system of nurse–client which is different from the interpersonal system of the family alone. The assessment process itself is therapeutic. As the nurse elicits and verifies the perceptions of the members, their awareness of self and of others is heightened. This interaction between nurse and client helps identify each member's concerns and problems. The nurse–therapist communicates his/her perception of the information shared and the behaviors observed with the family system. The reframing of this data by the therapist provides an alternative perspective which may or may not be acceptable to the individuals. When members' perceptions differ from those of the nurse, they are encouraged to voice their exceptions—demonstrating that it is all right to disagree. There is no potential for resolution unless dissension is openly expressed.

Once individual needs, values, and goals have been acknowledged, the family is assisted in looking for common ground. During this endeavor, the nurse emphasizes how the stress or problems one member is experiencing affects each of the other members and the family as a whole. It is important that while members learn to respect the individuality of one another, they maintain a sense of the family system. The nurse facilitates the interaction process as shared goals are established and means to achieve the same are negotiated so that members can assume responsibility (King, 1983).

Therapy provides a non-threatening environment in which family members can explore alternative modes of interaction. The nurse–therapist serves as educator, mediator, facilitator, and resource to the family. As members engage in goal-directed behavior leading to transactions, the health of the family system is promoted. The measure of therapeutic effectiveness is the family's ability to function as an interpersonal system—independent of the nurse–therapist—in a manner conducive to maintaining a state of health.

Case Example

The following data were gathered during the assessment process with the family system. The subsystems include:

- *Tom:* 49-year-old male; married to Donna for 11 months; one previous marriage, divorced 5 years; two adult children (male and female); stepfather to Gwen; employed full-time in retailing.
- *Donna:* 42-year-old female; widowed at age 28 when daughter (Gwen) was three years old; employed part-time, bookkeeper.

- *Gwen:* 17-year-old female; only natural child of Donna, father deceased; stepdaughter to Tom; senior in high school.

Perceptions of Concerns and Problems Presented by Family

Donna: Initiated contact with the nurse–therapist. Identifying Gwen as the problem, Donna has become increasingly disturbed by her daughter's behavior the last few months. Donna perceives Gwen as being argumentative, disrespectful, and irresponsible. Gwen has violated curfew, allowed her grade point average to drop, has become lax in keeping her room clean, and seems determined to disregard Donna's advice and defy her directives. Conversations with her daughter all turn into arguments. Donna does not understand what has happened to their relationship; "we used to be so close." The late father's pension allowed her to work only part-time so that she could be at home with Gwen as much as possible. "But, now, my presence seems to irritate her."

Donna does not feel that Tom has been supportive in dealing with Gwen. "Though he means well, he just doesn't know Gwen as I do. He doesn't recognize the change in her. He thinks that I'm overreacting, that I'm too hard on her." Donna really doesn't expect that Tom would understand, but she wishes he wouldn't interfere. For some reason, Tom thinks that if Donna were working full-time, she wouldn't worry so much about Gwen. He's also been after her to go out with him more in the evening, to a movie or to visit friends. "He should realize that Gwen needs my supervision now more than ever." Donna wonders if Gwen's friends have gotten her to experiment with drugs that have caused the change in her. "I don't know how else to explain it, or what to do. I'm at my rope's end."

Tom: Tom is experiencing both concern and frustration. He doesn't like to see Donna and Gwen arguing all the time. He doesn't doubt that they have a deep affection for one another, and he suggests it's just a phase they're going through. Tom perceives Donna as being overprotective, perhaps possessive, of Gwen. That's why he thinks Donna should consider going to work on a full-time basis. Tom reluctantly admits that he has, at times, felt like an outsider. Those are times when Donna dismisses any input he offers regarding Gwen. "After all, I've raised two children of my own, and would like to help Donna with Gwen. She really is a good kid."

Gwen: Gwen is of the opinion that there would be no problem if her mother would just "get off my case." She seems to think Tom agrees with her, even though he hasn't actually said so. Gwen perceives herself to be in a no-win situation with her mother. "One minute she's telling me that I'm old enough to accept responsibility for scheduling my activities to allow enough time for homework and preparing for tests. The next minute she's setting a curfew to make sure I'm home early enough to study and get the amount of rest she thinks I need. Or, then, I'm old enough to pick up after myself, that my room is my responsibility. But I can't put any posters on the wall or rearrange the furniture the way I like it. She says she's the adult and she makes those kinds of decisions." Gwen insists that neither she nor her circle of friends take drugs, though they may drink beer at a party. Gwen angrily poses the question: "If I'm old enough to accept all those responsibilities, why aren't

I old enough for her to trust me? She doesn't even give me a chance to make my own decisions. No matter what I do, I get in trouble with her. So I don't even care any more."

As the family members communicate their perceptions, the nurse–therapist observes the non-verbal behaviors. Facial expressions and voice tones are consistent with the content of their messages: Donna presents a greal deal of stress and exasperation; Tom presents concern and frustration; and Gwen presents bewilderment and anger. Donna looks at Gwen as Gwen is speaking, though she does not evidence similar interest in Tom's perceptions. Tom maintains eye contact with the nurse throughout the interaction process, while Gwen seeks to avoid any eye contact. As the members are sharing their perceptions, the nurse–therapist verifies the information as he/she is assessing and formulating diagnoses within the theoretical framework of the practice model.

Assessment

The altered health state of the family system is reflected in each family member in terms of social roles: Donna as parent and wife; Gwen as child and student; and Tom as stepfather and husband. The family's perceptions regarding the source of the present difficulties are not, however, congruent. Donna perceives Gwen to be the problem. Gwen, in reality, is struggling with tasks of developing from an adolescent to a young adult. These tasks include: evaluating her own limitations and powers; examining and anticipating the consequences of her own decisions; and critically evaluating ideals, beliefs, attitudes, and values (Peplau, 1951). Yet Gwen's mastery of this stage of development is experienced by Donna as a threat to her parental identity. Few roles are enacted with as much consistency as that of a single parent. It is understandable that Donna's parental role would have become so integrated into her sense of self that relinquishing the role could precipitate a crisis. Just as important, however, is Gwen's sense of self as she is attempting to bridge the gap between adolescence and young adulthood. For, as King notes (1981), the concept of self is reflected in patterns of growth and development within the interaction processes of the family system. Both Donna and Gwen are experiencing a maturational crisis as their parent–child relationship is undergoing redefinition. Donna is vascillating, for on some level she is aware of Gwen's developmental needs. Yet she does not want to "let go" of her child. Her energies are focused on maintaining the parental role, seemingly to the point of neglecting her newly acquired role of wife. Donna's ambivalence is evidenced in the contradictory messages she is giving Gwen. Although Gwen recognizes the contradictory communication, she is unable to escape the situation. The impact has extended to the suprasystem as her enactment of the student role is also affected. When Gwen acts out her confusion and anger, Donna's parental perceptions of her as a child are reinforced.

A vicious cycle ensues in which both are experiencing a great deal of stress.

As a member of the family system, Tom could provide support to Donna and Gwen. There are, however, incongruent expectations regarding Tom's role in the family. Donna seems to perceive her recent marriage as parallel to, though separate from, her relationship with her daughter. The perception is one of co-existing systems rather than interrelated subsystems comprising the family system. Donna's view does not allow for recognizing the relationship between Tom and Gwen as stepfather/stepdaughter. The only expectation Donna has of Tom in terms of Gwen is that he not interfere. She does, however, expect him to be supportive of her in the role of spouse. Tom, on the other hand, has more of a sense of being part of a family unit in which he is both husband and stepfather. He had expected to function in both roles and is willing to accept the responsibility of doing so. Out of frustration, his energies are centered upon the marriage in which his role is recognized. Having lost her natural father at an early age, Gwen is receptive to at least exploring Tom's role as a stepfather. She seems to be seeking an ally in Tom—hoping that he would somehow be able to rescue her from the situation with her mother.

DIAGNOSES

- Maturational crises as a result of rigid perceptions and ambiguous, contradictory communication.
- Incongruent role expectations related to perceptions not being shared and verified.
- Lack of integration of subsystems within the family system.

Intervention: Determination of Shared Goals

Having formulated diagnoses from the assessment data, the nurse–therapist shares his/her perceptions of the interactional processes with the family. The family members' reactions are elicited and they are encouraged to verify perceptions among themselves. Through open communication facilitated by the therapist, the family expresses needs, expectations, and goals. Each member of the nurse–client interpersonal system participates in determining those goals to which all are willing to direct their behaviors. The nurse coaches the interaction as means to achieve the established goals. In time, agreement is reached on the following goals and means:

- *Goal:* To support the maturational development of Gwen and Donna.
- *Means:* Verbalize perceptions of what the role transitions mean to each individual; discuss and explore developmental needs; provide support in mastering new tasks; concur upon expectations of changing roles.
- *Goal:* To convey clear, consistent messages.

- *Means:* Heighten awareness of verbal and nonverbal behavior; verify perceptions with one another; when ambiguity is observed, acknowledge and examine its source.
- *Goal:* To integrate Tom into the family system.
- *Means:* Identify the variety and interrelatedness of new roles—husband/wife, stepfather/stepdaughter; share perceptions and expectations of each role; seek congruence between role expectations and behaviors.

As members work together to accomplish goals, they learn to recognize and understand each other as individuals. Multiple interactions lead to trust and the resolution of problems (King, 1983). A sense of the family as a system of interrelationships is enhanced.

By engaging family resources to deal with stressors, members are better able to function in their social roles. Transactions are experienced. If the health of the family system is sustained following the termination of therapy—and the nurse–client interpersonal system—the intervention will have been effective.

SUMMARY

This chapter has presented a model of family therapy derived from King's conceptual framework and theory of goal attainment, as well as her formulations on family nursing (1981, 1983). The model is applicable to various family structures. The interpersonal system of the family is the focal system of the model. The personal systems of family members are the subsystems, and the environmental social systems comprise the familial suprasystem. Knowledge of both the individual members and the environment enhances understanding of the family. During the therapeutic process, the nurse enters into an interpersonal system with the family client. Assessment focuses on the perceptions, communications, roles, and developmental stages of members, as well as the stressors being experienced within the system. Through purposeful interaction, the nurse–therapist facilitates the process whereby family members establish shared goals and negotiate means to achieve them. As transactions occur, the health of the family system is promoted.

Potential avenues of inquiry into King's conceptual framework, the theory of goal, and this practice model are unlimited. Both deductive and inductive methodologies are warranted. The theory of goal attainment posits relationships between concepts of the model which need to be subjected to empirical tests. Examples of additional research questions are: How do different family system structures and compositions affect role expectations? Does the ratio of familial roles to extrafamilial roles (in the suprasystem) have an impact on the health of the family system? What factors in the nurse–client interpersonal system enhance or impede transactions? Such investigations would enhance the descriptive, explanatory, and predictive powers of King's theory of goal attainment and yield subsequent refinement of the practice model.

FOUR CENTRAL COMPONENTS OF NURSING APPROACHES

- **Title of Chapter:** Family Therapy as Derived from King's Conceptual Model
- **Definitions**
- **Family:** An interpersonal system of individuals interacting to meet basic needs through communication and perception of the internal and external environment.
- **Family Environment:** The interpersonal system of the family is the immediate social environment of the individual. The external environment is the suprasystem in which the family functions.
- **Family Health:** Dynamic life experiences through which the family adjusts to environmental stressors to achieve maximum potential for daily living. Family health is reflected in the members' abilities to function in social roles.
- **Therapist's Approach:** Forms an interpersonal system with the family and engages members in purposeful communication to determine shared goals and means to achieve them.

REFERENCES

Aguilera, D., & Messick, J. (1974). *Crisis intervention: Theory and methodology.* St. Louis: C. V. Mosby.

American Nurses' Association. (1973). *Standards of nursing practice.* Kansas City, Mo.: American Nurses' Association.

American Nurses' Association. (1976). *Code for nurses with interpretive statements.* Kansas City, Mo.: American Nurses' Association.

Barrell, L. (March 1974). Crisis intervention: Partnership in problem-solving. *Nursing Clinics of North America*, pp. 5–16.

Caplan, G. (1961). *An approach to community mental health.* New York: Grune & Stratton.

Glasser, P., & Glasser, L. (1970). Adequate family functioning. In P. Glasser & L. Glasser (Eds.), *Families in crisis.* New York: Harper & Row.

Gonot, P. J. (1983). Imogene M. King: A theory for nursing. In J. Fitzpatrick & A. Whall (Eds.), *Conceptual models of nursing: Analysis and application.* Bowie, Md.: Brady.

King. I. M. (1981). *A theory for nursing.* New York: Wiley.

King, I. M. (1983). King's theory of nursing. In I. Clements & F. Roberts (Eds.), *Family health: A theoretical approach to nursing care.* New York: Wiley.

Peplau, H. E. (1975). Foreword. In S. Smoyak (Ed.), *The psychiatric nurse as a family therapist.* New York: Wiley.

Peplau, H. E. (1951). *Tools and tasks outline.* Unpublished manuscript. Teachers College, Columbia University.

Williams, F. (1971). Maturational crises. *Perspectives in Psychiatric Care, 9* (6) pp. 240–246.

— APPROACH TWO

Use of a Nursing Model To Deductively Reformulate an Existing Family Therapy Theory

4

Strategic Family Therapy: Nursing Reformulations and Applications

Ann L. Whall

This chapter examines an existing family therapy theory, Madanes' (1981, 1984) strategic family therapy, in light of Roy's (1981, 1983, 1984) nursing model. Strategic family therapy as discussed by Jones, is described in Chapter 6 as being one of the interactionist approaches. In her discussion, Jones points out that there are many therapies found under the overall interactionist umbrella. Strategic family therapy, although not a new approach, has most recently been explicated by Madanes. Because it is one of the clearest presentations of this approach, the work of Madanes rather than that of other strategic family therapists is used in this chapter. Roy's model is used in this chapter because of the facility with which nursing interventions may be addressed within the model and because this same type of facility is found in Madanes' work. These two theoretical approaches also demonstrate other underlying compatibilities. Madanes, for example, presents an optimistic view in that change in a problematic family system is seen as not only possible but probable in light of certain approaches taken by the therapist. Roy presents this same optimistic view in that the nurse in Roy's model is seen as changing an existing system by certain types of actions. It is understood that Roy's model is more abstract than the practice theory of Madanes and this is seen as quite helpful. That is, Roy's model may be used as an overall guide from which to view strategic therapy. Where commonalities are found, these may be strengthened or further elaborated using Roy's model. When differences are found, Roy's model may be and is used as a guide to change strategic family therapy.

Entire sets of statements and concepts are taken from the strategic theory and viewed from Roy's model. The statements and concepts selected are those which concern nursing's four central concepts: person/family, environment, health, and nursing. Propositions and concepts were left unchanged where possible. When this was not possible the statements and concepts were changed so as to be compatible with Roy. Two types of criteria were used to make the judgment "goodness of fit," or congruency. The first criterion was the assessment of strategic theory and Roy's model in terms of the types of concepts and statements used. That is, Roy's model and strategic family therapy were viewed in terms of the use of organismic and mechanistic concepts and relationships which related to the four central concepts of nursing. Secondly, the assumptions of strategic therapy were identified where possible and examined for congruency with Roy. When these statements would lead to actions that would appear conflictual with Roy, these were changed so as to be more consistent with Roy. This process is similar to the theory derivation process described by Walker and Avant (1983). Inferences needed to be made in terms of practice approaches derived from Roy's model, but then in all practice situations this needs to be done. The validity of these inferences can be established by continual reexamination of Roy's model.

This chapter first identifies similarities between Roy's and Madanes' approaches. Then strategic family therapy is examined in terms of discussions relating to the environment, family health, family unit, the role of the therapist, and the healing process. Roy's model is then examined for the same elements and the reformulated approach is presented. A case example follows with application of the reformulated nursing approach.

STRATEGIC FAMILY THERAPY: SIMILARITY TO ROY'S MODEL

In a discussion of the elements of strategic family therapy, Madanes (1981) identified as a feature of strategic family therapy the belief that the therapist must plan a strategy to approach the family's problem. In addition, the therapist is to identify the interactional or family organizational structure associated with the problem; prescribe certain types of directives; and identify the underlying metaphor expressed by the family problem.

In a similar view, Roy (1983) has the nurse assess the family's survival or continuity needs; growth and self-concept needs; transactional and interdependence patterns; and member control and role factors. Roy says that assessment does not stop at this point, but that the nurse also looks at the way in which the focal, contextual, and residual stimuli are related.

The similarities in both approaches lie in the nurse or therapist being active or directive, the assessments being related to the presenting problem, and behaviors being clustered together in order to understand the problem. Madanes looked for the analogue of the problem behavior (i.e., considering the problem to be analogous to some aspect of family functioning). In both strategic family therapy and Roy's approach, the therapist sets goals with the family and gives directives concerning the problem. Although Roy does not specifically discuss looking for analogy in behavior, the fact that the nurse examines the context of the presenting problem or stimuli would lead to examination of similarities between the presenting problem and the total family situation. Directives from Roy's perspective would be handled by setting goals based on the family's input. That is, the directives would be related to the mutual goals or, if formulated by the nurse alone, would be derived from these goals. In summary, both approaches appear optimistic, goal-directed, intervener active, and contextually focused. The approaches are both optimistic in that it is anticipated that change can and will likely occur if goals are set and directives are carried out. The intervener in both approaches clearly takes the initiative in assessing the family. Neither approach would suggest the "blank screen" of other therapies, that is, in both approaches, questions are asked and prescriptions given. Both approaches also consider the context of the problem, or in Roy's terms, the contextual stimuli.

The existing approach which is modified for nursing (i.e., strategic family therapy) is presented first in terms of family environment external to the family, family health, role of the therapist, and family unit conceptualization.

ENVIRONMENT, FAMILY, FAMILY HEALTH, ROLE OF THERAPIST

The Strategic Approach

The environment of the family for Madanes (1981, 1984) appears to be a separate but approachable and potentially helpful resource. The therapist, for example, seeks out a vocational guidance agency to assist a woman once the problem is defined as poor self-concept. Environment in strategic family therapy is seen as the context in which the family exists and in which the symptoms arise. Roy has defined the term environment, whereas Madanes has not specifically done so. Roy and Roberts (1981) stated that the term *environment* is defined in the dictionary as the conditions surrounding persons which affect the development and behavior of an organism or a group of organisms. This definition appears to be compatible with that of the strategic approach. That is, the environment of the family may be their home, their friends, their neighborhood, the air they breathe, and food they eat. In the view of both approaches, persons as well as social and physical systems are the environment of the family.

Family health, or the optimal state sought by the therapist, must be inferred in the strategic approach for it is not discussed directly by Madanes. Many of Madanes' case examples regarding healthy family functioning have to do with organizational clarity and competence. Cross-generational coalitions cause a lack of clarity in the family system. This lack of clarity is seen as non-healthy, for it leads to symptomatic behavior on the part of children. In addition, two other theorists from this school, Haley (1978) and Minuchin (1974), discuss family health as related to balanced relationships between subsystems (i.e., parents and children). The balance at certain times is unequal, however, as when children are young or when a family member is ill. A lack of balance between members within a subsystem (for example, husbands and wives) also appears to be non-healthy for it leads to many struggles, both overt and covert. Competence, or taking responsibility for actions, appears to be healthy for all subsystems within the family. In multiple examples, Madanes presented problem behavior of children as a manifestation of a problem between the parents. As this "acting out" is in essence non-healthy, a healthy family would not have members who are "acting out," but ones who are free to grow, not bound by symptoms of other members. Family health in strategic family therapy, therefore, concerns interactional patterns. In summary, family health in strategic family therapy is manifested by a balancing of negotiation patterns, organizational clarity and competence, and a freedom for individuals and subsystems to grow and develop, unfettered by constricting alliances.

The role of the family therapist in Madanes' approach is quite clear. The therapist is in charge of the therapy and the therapy is focused around the presenting problem. The therapist assesses the metaphorical actions enacted by the family around the problem. The therapist is an enabler of change in family behavior. Often techniques are used such as "pretending" in which a type of paradox is used. That is, the family may be asked to "pretend" a symptom, because a symptom "pretended" cannot be "real." As the therapist changes the context of the presenting symptom, there is a somewhat covert element to the therapy when the purpose of directives are not revealed to the client. A husband might be told to spend time "pretending" he comforts his bulemic wife whenever she vomits (Madanes, 1981). This action by the husband changes the effect of the symptom (i.e., the vomiting may no longer annoy or upset him). When the husband pretends to console his wife, he must give her attention and refrain at least while doing so from criticizing her. The directions for change, or the directives, thus center around changing the context of the problem. The context or situation in which the bulemia has been occurring has thus changed.

The family in strategic family therapy is approached as a unit, or as a whole. Another way of saying this is that in strategic family therapy the family is seen as a system. One consequence of approaching the family as a system is that problems are seen as originating within the system and not within individuals. Problems are seen as originating in the context of the total interactional pattern of all family members. An individual family member, therefore, does not have a problem—the family unit or system has a problem. This is not an additive approach, it is a holistic approach focused upon the whole family system, not a group of individuals.

In this regard, the therapist focuses upon the present family—not upon the past—nor is a detailed family history taken. There is no attempt to solve problems from the past—this approach has been described as "ahistoric."

Oftentimes, however, a particular dyadic relationship in the family will be focused upon as being the most troublesome. This does not negate a holistic approach, because the entire unit is considered, and all relationships are evaluated before this focus occurs. Within a unitary conceptualization of the family, a change in one portion of the family system will have an effect upon, and in essence change, the entire system.

The "healing process" or therapy is the way in which the therapist goes about working with the family, so that a more "healthy" state may be achieved. In strategic family therapy, "the emphasis is not upon a method to be applied in all cases" (Madanes, 1981, p. 19) but rather upon designing a specific approach to a given problem. There is also an emphasis upon developmental stages of persons and families. The healing process is therefore focused upon assisting the family "past a crisis" (Madanes, 1981, p. 20) and on to the next developmental stage.

In the strategic approach, problems that exist in the family are seen as adaptive to a particular situation. The therapist has the task, according to Madanes, of framing the problem in solvable terms (1981). The therapist often proceeds to introduce alternative patterns or alternative ways of behaving (1981). The therapist introduces steps or plans steps for the family to take that may reestablish certain organizational patterns within the family system (1981). The therapist "motivates" (1981, p. 24) the family to follow through on directives, sometimes using personal influence in discussions. Madanes summarizes in essence the therapeutic strategies to be used during the healing process in this way: approaches are devised to address the organizational structure of the family, to address hierarchies of incompatible power structures, and to focus upon understanding the metaphor expressed by the symptom (1981).

The therapist joins or experiences the family system in order to understand the system. At the same time, the therapist maintains a detached perspective that aids in assessment and in intervention. The family is seen as unaware of the metaphor underlying the situation. In this view, calling the family's attention directly to the metaphor would do little to change the situation. Rather, the family is caught as it were in a repetitious attempt to solve the problem. Information alone is seen as unlikely to bring about change. The therapist changes the context of the problem so that unsuccessful attempts are diverted. The family is then able to experience a new way of handling the situation.

Roy's Approach

Since the initial statements regarding the adaption model, Sister Callista Roy has continued to discuss, develop, and extend the model (Roy, 1971, 1976, 1981, 1983, 1984). Because nursing models often have not attempted to address the family as a unit of analysis, it is particularly helpful when theorists make this application. Roy (1983) has done so, and her discussions of the application of the model to families are used as a basis for the following discussion. Roy (1981) said that the client may be a person, a family, a group, or a community. In Roy's view practice theory is one logical outcome in terms of her model; a family may be the primary focus of the nurse, and assisting troubled families is an acceptable activity for nursing.

Roy's model identifies the recipient of nursing care as an adaptive system (1981), and because the family is an adaptive system it is seen as a proper recipient of care. Adaptive responses are those that promote integrity in terms of survival, growth, reproduction, and self-mastery (1981). Adaptive responses for the family in this view would promote the survival of the family, would support the growth and development of individual members and the overall system, and would enable the family to master tasks such as successful negotiations with outside systems.

Roy has stated that the family can be thought of as an adaptive system (1981). The family is thus described as "acting to maintain itself in regard to the four modes" (Roy, 1981, p. 43), i.e., physiologic, self-concept, role function, and interdependence. (See Fig. 4–1.) Roy discussed the internal "processor systems" of persons as the cognator and regulator. These systems function in relation to the four modes. One may think of the four modes as ways in which families seek integrity, growth, reproduction, and self-mastery, and of the cognator and regulator systems as processes used in these attempts.

Roy (1976) stated that a given stimulus may fall beyond an individual's adaptative range; when this happens the person repeatedly and unsuccessfully attempts to cope. The nurse in Roy's model assesses these attempts to cope. A second-level assessment is made of the focal, contextual, and residual stimuli.

A nurse–therapist therefore assesses the family's attempt to adapt in terms of the four modes and also assesses the stimuli. The focal stimulus is the stimulus most immediately confronting the family (Roy, 1981). For example, the retirement of the primary wage earner in the family could be seen as a focal stimulus. Contextual stimuli would in this instance be all other stimuli present in the situation (e.g., the fact that the family rents their home). Residual stimuli are background factors such as "beliefs, attitudes, experiences, or traits" (Roy, 1981, p. 55). In terms of this example, beliefs that the family needs to be active socially would be seen as residual stimuli.

Roy discussed the family as a focus of her model in later works (1983, 1984). In terms of the conceptualization of family, Roy indeed uses a unitary approach. That is, the family is seen as a system to be viewed in terms of input (or stimuli) and output (or adaptive as well as nonadaptive responses). Roy, therefore, does not view the family as a collection of individuals

Roy (1983, p. 269) defined health as "a state and process of being and becoming an integrative whole person." Since persons as well as families are referred to as systems it would seem that a healthy family system is one which is integrated and whole. In addition, Roy discussed high-level wellness, an example of which is awareness and responsibility, as well as sensitivity to other human beings. A healthy family, therefore, would be aware and responsible in terms of individual needs and one in which roles are complementary.

The therapist in Roy's model would be active in the management of stimuli, in order to bring these stimuli within the adaptive range. Family support might be sought to help the family live within a diminished income. The context of the problem would be evaluated so as to identify

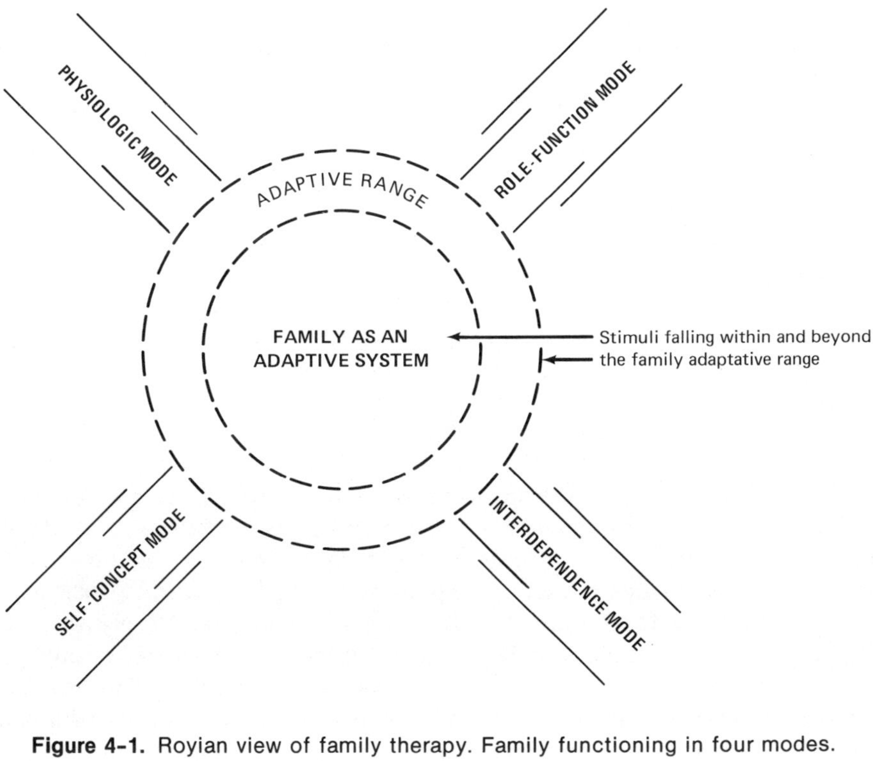

Figure 4-1. Royian view of family therapy. Family functioning in four modes.

the most troublesome areas. Once the contextual stimulus that was most troublesome was identified, it would either be changed, avoided, or altered in some way. Renting a smaller, more affordable home when finances are inadequate might be one change which could be fostered. Residual stimuli such as beliefs might be addressed by the therapist so as to change the stimuli. Beliefs that the family might hold (i.e., unreal expectations) could be addressed.

Before management of the stimuli, however, the therapist would first assess the four adaptive modes of the family. For example, physiologic needs, self-concept, role function, and interdependence would be assessed. Disturbances in these modes (i.e., the ways in which the family was meeting its food, clothing, shelter, and activity needs) would be important. Roy has stated that for the personal self, self-consistency, self-ideal, and self-esteem are important aspects of the self concept system (1981, p. 250). Difficulties or disturbances in these areas would be identified. Roy further stated that the self-concept system serves to meet the basic need of psychic integrity as well as to promote adaptation (1981).

Roy used Malaznik's definition of role function (1981). Role function is the expected behaviors that the person should perform to maintain a title. Family difficulties would be manifested in terms of carrying out family roles (e.g., financial support). The interdependence adaptive mode according to Roy is manifested by a balance in relationships with others (1983). Interdependence is related to the need for affection and nurturing. The family is assessed in terms of this mode and of related symptoms. The family may not, for example, be nurturing one another because of the crisis over financial matters.

Finally, nursing intervention in Roy's model can be viewed as directing the healing process. Roy stated that the client is an adaptive system, and the goal of adaptation is to bring the focal stimuli within the adaptive change. Nursing intervention thus focuses on managing the focal contextual and residual stimuli so that coping takes place. Thus the stimuli, the adaptive modes, and the adaptive range are all taken into consideration.

In the healing process the nurse "examines the contextual and residual stimuli associated with the focal stimulus, to ascertain the zone within which family coping can take place" (Roy, 1983, p. 276) and to identify the stimulus outside the zone which will require intervention. Based on the assessment, the nurse identifies related nursing diagnoses with related goals and interventions (Roy, 1983). In the healing process the nurse assists the family so that they can deal more effectively with the situation. From a Royian viewpoint, the nurse assesses the family, develops a nursing diagnosis, and sets related goals and interventions. The goals appear to be mutually set and the interventions shared at least as far as possible with the family.

CONGRUENCE AND REFORMULATION

The examination for congruence, or goodness of fit, between strategic family therapy and Roy's approach is organized in the following manner. First, there is identification of the four central concepts, expanded to include conceptualizations of family unit, family health, environment external to the family, and role of the therapist. As these areas are examined, questions are asked regarding the nature of concepts and relationships. In terms of the four family therapy concepts, questions are asked regarding the assumptions and the action statements found in the two approaches. Finally, suggestions are made for reformulation of the strategic family therapy.

In terms of the conceptualization of the family unit, both the strategic approach and Roy use a systems perspective. The family is seen as a system and approached as a whole. There is consistency between the two approaches on this point. In terms of either approach, both use a systems perspective which appears more organismic than mechanistic.

Family health definitions were inferred from both discussions. Strategic therapy in essence considers family health to be related to organizational clarity and competence. In this view family members should be free to grow and change. In Roy's model family health was seen as awareness and responsibility, as integration of roles and a concern by family members for the family. A similarity appears in the area of concern for individual needs and a balancing of these rights with those of the family as a whole. Role clarity and competence of family members in their roles also appear important in both approaches. Thus the inferred definitions of family health appear to be compatible. Moreover because of the holistic emphasis, they appear more organismic than mechanistic.

The environment external to the family also appears congruent in both approaches: the environment is all that is external to family. The environment is seen as potentially helpful—not a negative factor. The definitions of environment in both approaches do not appear mechanistic, with one exception. If both approaches are inferred to conceive of the environment as totally separate from families, rather than as co-extensive, the approach might be described as mechanistic. It is not clear that this is the case, however.

In terms of the therapist's approach it seems that the assessment phases would differ. Roy would address the ways in which the identified problem was affecting the four adaptive modes of the family. A second assessment would be of the focal contextural and residual stimuli. The nurse would assess these with the input of the family. The adaptive range would also be evaluated. Thus Roy appears to give more guidelines for the assessment process.

The diagnosis, which Roy indicates is needed, would flow from Roy's assessment process. In the reformulation effort, strategic terms could be in this process. Thus, from Roy's approach the family would assist in evaluation of the problem but strategic therapy terms would be used in this effort. A diagnosis might be, for example, a disturbance in the self-concept mode of the parents and a metaphorical acting out on the part of a child.

One difference in the two approaches is that Roy's approach includes a history. Roy stated the nurse would ask "what is the history of support and nurturance in this family?" (Roy, 1983, p. 302). She added that the history of the family as an adaptive system is very important. This emphasis is contrasted with the "ahistoric" approach of strategic therapy.

In Roy's model the healing process or intervention might involve techniques such as role playing and the discussion of opinions (Roy, 1983). Similar interventions could be derived from the strategic approach. For example, the strategic therapy seeks as a goal clear organizational structure and role competence. These goals are related to Roy's goals concerning role adaptation. The interventions described by Madanes could thus be used (e.g., "trying out" and "pretending"). In summary, goals and interventions suggested by strategic therapy would each be examined for usefulness with Roy. Evaluation of the therapy would proceed on the basis of the attainment of goals.

What are the differences? Roy provides multiple assessment parameters, for example, history taking and mutual goal setting. The strategic approach on the other hand provides fewer assessment categories and more techniques for intervention. Finally, Roy considers the physiologic needs of individuals and families and this is not as evident in the strategic approach. The assumptions of Roy appear to be that the family is capable of change, willing to change, and in need of assistance in terms of the focal stimuli. Strategic family therapy also assumes the capability and willingness of the family to change, but approaches the change in a somewhat less direct fashion. An assumption of this latter approach may be that much of what motivates behavior is not consciously available to family members. Besides this difference in conscious motivation there is also a difference in terms of covert approaches that the therapist uses. Roy's approach uses fewer of these covert approaches and more of a mutually shared (with the family) approach.

The reformulated approach is applied in the hypothetical case example below. As stated at the outset of this chapter, entire sets of statements were taken from strategic family therapy and viewed from Roy's model in order to develop the reformulated approach. The statements selected were those which concerned nursing's four central concepts: person, environment, health, and nursing. These concepts were identified in both the strategic approach and Roy's approach in terms of the view of family, family environment, family health (or the goal of therapy), and the role of the therapist or nurse. Inherent in the role of therapist are assessment and intervention strategies. When the strategic approach was found congruent with Roy, statements regarding these four concepts were left unchanged. When these statements were not found compatible with Roy they were changed so as to be compatible.

Case Example

For this family with a 32-year-old mother, Suzie, the presenting problem is that about 6 months ago the father, Mike, died very suddenly. About 6 months later, Suzie began what can be termed "acting out." That is, in a non-stop marathonlike fashion, Suzie began staying out all night, not cooking, drinking very heavily and in general not caring for the children or the home. The children, Sarah, Tim, and John, ages 13, 11, and 7, have been paying the bills, cleaning, and attempting to keep the house and family going. Because of their inexperience, things are not going well. They often oversleep and are late for school because of the mother's "carrying on" all night at home with men friends or the necessity to stay awake to help her get drunkenly into bed.

Suzie has few if any extended family members, as she is an only child. Her husband, Mike, a successful account executive, left the family financially well off and the family continues to live a life-style which may be termed "upper middle class." Mike's family are remote to this family unit, having not approved of the marriage of their son to Suzie, a 19-year-old at the time and not a college graduate. Mike died of a heart attack at age 42. At the time the family had moved to a new state; consequently the family have few friends or acquaintances to rely upon.

The school authorities reported the family to protective services, whereupon the mother went for individual psychotherapy. She was placed on lithium, which she took only sporadically. She continued to drink on occasion to excess, and in general did not alter her behavior. The children were not seen in individual therapy but their care, which improved only somewhat, was monitored by protective services.

At first it seemed to the nurse–therapist that the diagnosis of manic depressive disorder for the mother was indeed correct. As correct as this medical diagnosis appeared, the treatment was ineffective, however, even after the hospitalizations of Suzie. From the perspective presented here, the treatment was ineffective because the assessment was lacking. The terms from Roy's model are used for this assessment as are compatible strategic therapy terms. The focal stimuli, in terms of adaptation of the family unit, was the death of the father and the seeming inability of the mother to function without the father. The nurse proceeded to analyze the contextual and residual stimuli. The contextual stimulus is primarily that as the mother acted incompetently, the children acted as parents to the mother and did so in a more or less competent fashion. The oldest daughter, Sarah, now acted as the primary caregiver in the family. She was, however, continually castigated by Suzie. John was showing immature behavior, crying continually and refusing to leave his mother's side. He even slept in his mother's room. The other children did not appear to respond at first to their father's death, perhaps because of the need not to show signs of grief to the mother.

The residual stimuli presented essential information for the understanding of the focal stimuli. The mother, Suzie, an only child, was born to her parents when her mother, Marilyn, was 42 and her father, Frank, was 52. Suzie's mother could be described as a socialite, having been born to poverty and later marrying Frank, a man of wealth. Well respected in an upper middle class community, trouble occurred when Frank was 65, Marilyn 55, and Suzie 13. Frank's company changed ownership, Frank went "on his own," and lost most of the family wealth, as well as his pension money and the family home, while attempting to make a success of his own company. Marilyn was frantic, with poverty looming in the future as a shadow of the past. Using the remaining family wealth, Marilyn began a "flight into life," i.e., holding nonstop parties held in a frantic attempt to deny poverty, deny retirement without funds, and even deny the possibility of death. Frank almost totally ignored his family, throwing himself full time into his new job. Suzie, at entry into adolescence, was ignored by the party-giving mother and the preoccupied father. Meals were not prepared, housework not done, and the bills not paid.

Suzie became ill at age 14 and was hospitalized for a non-specific physical illness. The mother dropped her party-giving behavior and began caring for Suzie, staying at the hospital 24 hours a day, but only until Suzie came home. Then the "flight into life" continued, with her behavior as before.

In terms of reconceptualizing the therapy theory from a nursing perspective the hypothetical case example is used to demonstrate how the reformulated approach might be handled.

THE ASSESSMENT

The assessment categories that follow are those of Roy and compatible terms from strategic therapy. The focal stimuli are the death of the father, Mike, and the inability of the family to carry on without him. The death was falling outside of the adaptive range of the family and in a sense this was triggering off in the mother old, learned, non-adaptive responses, the flight into life. The residual stimuli provided needed data to understand the frantic activities of the mother. The children, try as they might, could not provide the needed overall family adaptation. Suzie's behavior was seen as a metaphor of the behavior she had witnessed in her family of origin, and this assessment uses a strategic therapy term. This analysis does not deny a physiologic link to behavior for as the nurse assessed the physiologic adaptive mode of Roy, the possibility that the crisis triggered off what might be called a "manic" physiologic behavior was possible. In terms of lithium for the mother, this might be seen as one method of bringing about an adaptation in this mode for the mother and thereby might assist in adaptation of the family.

In terms of the interdependence mode, the mother had few if any persons to rely upon except the children who were also feeling unnurtured.

This circularity in effect made adaptation almost impossible. The mother, or the parental subsystem, is seen as having a disturbance in both of the above adaptation modes of self-concept physiology and interdependence. The children subsystem was seen as having a problem with interdependence and self-concept. Their roles were age-inappropriate, their nurturance was in deficit, and at times not even their physiologic needs were being met. The family therefore showed disturbance in all four adaptive modes.

THE DIAGNOSIS AND INTERVENTION

The intervention approaches are those from Roy as well as those from strategic therapy that were found congruent with Roy's model. This family is having difficulty adapting to loss of a member, in large part owing to the past learning experience the mother had received in her family of origin and perhaps also to some physiologic response to a threatening crisis. In terms of strategic family therapy concepts, this family has an inverted organizational structure with the children acting as parents in terms of the overall family functioning and in terms of caring for Suzie as a parent would.

Suzie's activities and actions are metaphorically similar to those of her mother, Marilyn. As Marilyn faced loss and death she became an incompetent parent. When Suzie faced loss and death she also became an incompetent parent. Marilyn's flight into party giving was similar to Suzie's flight into drinking and "bar hopping." Moreover, Suzie had learned when she was 14, that when you are ill you are nurtured, when you are not ill you are not nurtured. Suzie was teaching her children this same lesson.

The analysis of the content of the situation is both from Roy (contextual stimuli) and strategic therapy. The context of Suzie's acting out is that, as the children try to "save" her, their added attention is a metaphor for the attention she didn't receive from her mother and later from her husband when he died. The clustering of the behavior together from the past and the present identified the major problem as being larger than the death of the husband and father. The organizational clarity of the family is non-existent as is role functioning and interdependence in terms of Roy's model. The children are acting as parents and the parent is acting like a child. Exactly who is to do what is not clear. Because the mother does not assume her role, the children's developmental needs (e.g., the need to be children) and thus the interdependence mode are not being met.

This analysis using Roy's and Madanes' terms focuses upon the interrelationship of family members, not upon Suzie. The children, except for Tim, are beginning to show signs of problems. Sarah is tearful and "nervous" most of the time, and it is not known if this is a pattern of withdrawal. Tim, however, spends long hours in his room alone, and John clings to his mother at every possible moment. The focal stimulus for the family, the death of the father, is thus being manifested in difficulty in Roy's adaptive modes interdependence role-function, in physiology, and in self-concept. The difficulty is also manifest in compatible concepts drawn from strategic therapy: that of lack of competence in the parental subsystem and an inverted organizational structure.

Before beginning the discussion of the healing process or therapeutic intervention, a review of the reformulated intervention approach may be helpful. The intervention goals according to Roy are responsibility in family roles and sensitivity to each other's needs. Adaptive responses are those that support the family's integrity, growth, and self-mastery. The context of the presenting stimulus or problem needs to be changed in order for change to occur toward these goals. The plan is to make it possible for the family to change its response pattern to losses. A discussion of this goal and assessment would be conducted with the family's input and agreement.

To meet Suzie's need for interdependence, a housekeeper could be engaged for the next year so that the mother could get back to her adult activities, such as returning to college. College might meet some of her self-concept needs and the housekeeper could assist with the interdependence needs. This would change the context of the family's presenting problem: loss of the competent father. It was determined that Suzie's acting as a child in need of nurturing needed to be "pretended." In light of this, Suzie might be directed to "pretend" for 2 hours each day that she is very ill, to lie on the couch, not to move, and to have her every need attended to by the children and the housekeeper. Suzie would thereby teach the children to be more competent. This also would meet Suzie's need for nurturing and attention. The children in turn might be given a directive—they are each to engage in at least one outside activity for 1 hour each day. They could do so as a group, or singly, but in no case could Suzie go along. This would teach the children to be competent in decision making and also would give Suzie a rest.

In this intervention, portions of the Roy approach are combined with compatible intervention portions of Madanes. Because of a need for a competent parent (Roy's role functioning) Suzie "pretends" to be incompetent. Because something "pretended" cannot be "real," this intervention changes the problematic role functioning in this family. The role-functioning changes indicated by Roy's model are approached, using a compatible portion of the strategic therapy approach. Teaching interventions are also suggested by Roy's model.

In order to change the contextual and residual stimuli so that the focal stimuli would fall within the family's adaptive range, family discussions might be held. Such discussions are suggested by Roy's model. The family would be apprised of the assessed needs. The goal of discussion is to review Suzie's experience as a child. The pros and cons of various adaptations to loss in her family of origin would be reviewed for and with the entire family. Underlying assumptions of Suzie's parents and how these affected this family would be identified. This intervention would seek to influence the residual stimuli or beliefs of this family.

As Suzie began taking her lithium regularly, she would become able to discuss these issues in these family sessions in a calmer fashion. Physiologic interventions are suggested by Roy's model but not, however, by strategic therapy. The context of the overall family response pattern and their subsequent involvement with protective services was, therefore, "reframed." The family was seen as in need of a "time out" to reexamine their needs, to take time to change their patterns. The death of Mike was reviewed and their feelings toward and about him discussed, both to dispel misperceptions and to relieve their anxiety and sorrow. The portion of these last interventions which are based upon Roy are teaching, discussing, and manipulating stimuli. The reframing is suggested by strategic therapy.

The response of this family is also hypothetical. Gradually the family would begin to function in a clearer organizational fashion. The inverted role structures would be changed. Because of the family's need for nurturing, the therapist would be aware that dependence could be a problem both in terms of the therapist and the housekeeper. Through changing the context (both Roy and Madanes suggest this) and using the educative approach, gradually the response to the major loss would be changed. Constructive, role-responsible, family behavior was the goal derived from both models. The interventions were aimed at this goal and therapy would be evaluated on this basis and changes made as needed.

The research needed upon this approach is evident. Do the two approaches blend in application? What are the consequences of a straightforward educative approach with an emotional response? Are the contextual changes effective in practice? There are multiple other questions that need to be asked both in practice and through research. In summary, strategic family therapy has been reformulated through the use of Roy's conceptual model. Areas of congruence were found between the two models. Roy's approach, however, would indicate a more informed participation on the part of the family. In Roy's approach, history of Suzie's experiences in her family of origin is important in understanding the current family situation.

RESEARCH AND EVALUATION

Theory developed for nursing practice must be evaluated in the real world. Oftentimes, however, it is assumed that research is the first step needed in this evaluation. Certainly research is a major and important way in which to examine, expand, change, or decide to discard theories, but it is not the only way or always the first step in this process. A discussion of Meleis (1985) regarding theory development may be helpful in clarifying this position. Meleis stated that there is a cycle in the process of theory development which includes these steps: practice—theory—research—theory—practice. Subportions of this cycle may be addressed in a theory development effort or, in this view, the cycle may be broken down into intermediate steps. For example—theory then practice and theory—may be addressed before research is undertaken.

This chapter began with theory, that of strategic therapy and Roy's model. The process began with theory and it is now suggested that the product of this theory discussion be examined in practice and, after analysis, that the theory be changed as necessary before research is addressed. In this view, partial theory should be more fully developed because the relationships posited are tentative and at times unclear. Once the relationships are more fully understood and developed, research may be undertaken.

In Meleis' schema, only step one in the theory/practice/theory process has been addressed in this chapter. That is, Roy's model was used to reformulate an existing therapy approach. Examples of the use of the reformulated approach in practice were described. In the next stage of this effort, the theory would be tried out in practice and necessary modifications made. Once this second step has taken place, research could address various relationships within the model or the model could be examined again in practice. In other words, practice evaluation would precede formal testing.

One might ask, what about the ethics of this? Is it not unethical to test out untried theories before research on the model is completed? These are rather naive questions, for in reality many of the more popular therapy theories are not well researched and in essence were developed via the theory—practice—theory route, although this may not have been well recognized. Discussion of research therefore is not addressed here; if these theoretical formulations prove useful, research must follow upon these theoretical efforts.

FOUR CENTRAL COMPONENTS OF NURSING APPROACHES

- **Title of Chapter:** Strategic Family Therapy: Nursing Reformulations and Applications
- **Definitions**
- **Family:** An adaptive system which is active and the recipient of care. Adaptive responses promote survival in four modes, physiologic, self-concept, role function, and interdependence.

- **Family Environment:** All that is external to the family; a potentially helpful factor (Roy, 1983).
- **Family Health:** An integrated and whole system; one which is able to adapt to stimuli with or without assistance.
- **Therapist's Approach:** Participative with or joins the family in terms of mutual goal setting. Assesses four modes and stimuli, helps to manage the stimuli to bring them within the family's adaptive range.

REFERENCES

Haley J. (1978). *Problem solving therapy.* San Francisco: Jossey Bass.

Madanes, C. (1981). *Strategic family therapy.* San Francisco: Jossey Bass.

Madanes, C. (1984). *Behind the one way mirror.* San Francisco: Jossey Bass.

Meleis, A. (1985). *Theoretical nursing: Development and progress.* Philadelphia: Lippincott.

Minuchin, S. (1974). *Families and family therapy.* Cambridge, Mass.: Harvard University Press.

Roy, C. (1971). Adaptation: A basis for nursing practice. *Nursing Outlook, 23,* 90–94.

Roy, C. (1976). *Introduction to nursing: An adaptation model.* Englewood Cliffs, N.J.: Prentice-Hall.

Roy, C. (1983). The Roy adaptation model. In I. Clements & F. Roberts (Eds.), *Family health: A theoretical approach to nursing care.* New York: Wiley.

Roy, C. (1984). *Introduction to nursing: An adaptation model.* (2nd ed.). Englewood Cliffs, N.J.: Prentice-Hall.

Roy, C., & Roberts, S. (1981). *Theory construction in nursing.* Englewood Cliffs, N.J.: Prentice-Hall.

Walker, L., & Avant, K. (1983). *Strategies for theory construction in nursing.* Norwalk, Conn.: Appleton-Century-Crofts.

5

The Developmental Conceptual Framework: Nursing Reformulations and Applications for Family Therapy

Pamela G. Reed

The family development conceptual model is a useful framework for construction of family theory and family therapy approaches in nursing. Developmental concepts are integral to nursing's understanding about human health and functioning (Newman, 1979; Parse, 1981; Rogers, 1970, 1980) of individuals, groups, families, and communities. Although not a family therapy model per se, the developmental framework provides a unique perspective for formulating family assessment and intervention. There is a great deal of similarity between the family development framework and Rogers' (1970, 1980) nursing conceptual model. Rogers' model is a conceptualization of the developmental processes of the human system. A nursing perspective of family development necessitates, however, some minor reformulations in the framework. Thus, this chapter addresses the deductive reformulation of the family development framework and its application to practice using Rogers' (1970, 1980) conceptual model.

THE FRAMEWORK

The family development framework evolved out of sociological perspectives on family functions and members' roles and psychological perspectives on individual developmental tasks and interpersonal interactions. Unique to this framework is its focus upon the longitudinal career of the family, i.e., the historical, social, and individual time dimensions in family life. Historical time refers to major political and economic events that occur during a family's lifespan; social time addresses those societal factors that are prevalent and influence family life; individual time represents the growth and developmental changes of an individual member as it affects family interrelationships. Family behavior is assumed to be a function of its past as well as present and cannot be understood without knowledge of ongoing developmental processes of the members (Hill, 1970).

Definition of Basic Concepts

The following diagram (Fig. 5–1) illustrates the framework's basic concepts and their organization. The concepts derive from a variety of sources

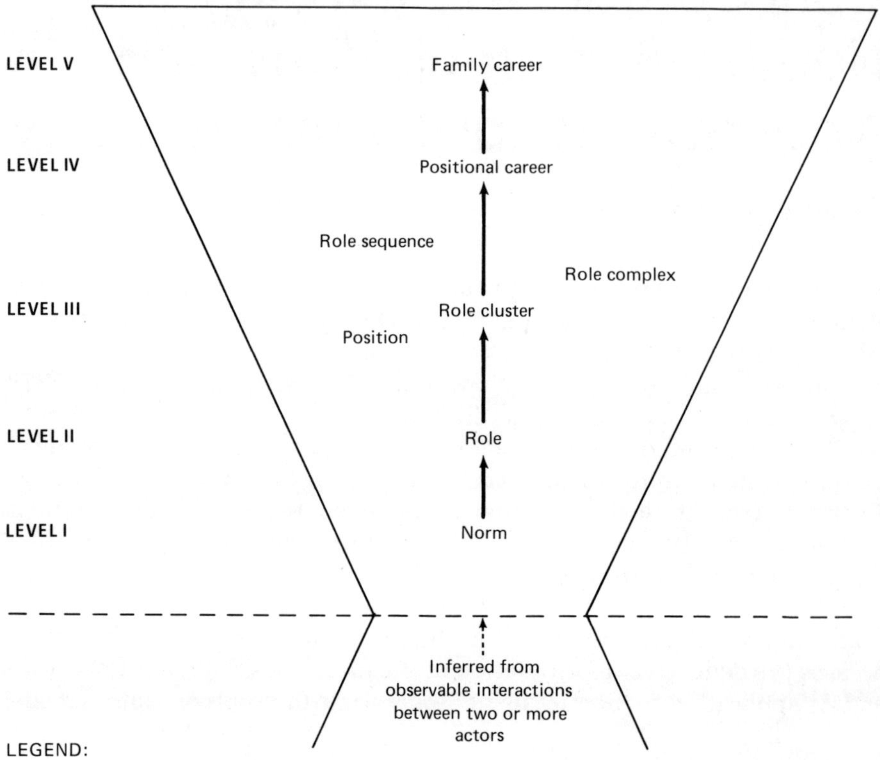

LEGEND:

Norm: A commonly held behavioral expectation
Role: Behaviors associated with a set of related norms
Position: The location of a person within a family system in relation to others and involving reciprocal sets of roles
Role cluster: The set of roles which make up a position at a given point in time
Role complex: The interactions of role clusters of two or more positions at a given point in time
Role sequence: The pattern of changes in roles that occurs over time, a series of roles
Positional career: The pattern of changes in sets of role clusters over time, i.e., the lifespan of an individual member
Family career: The pattern of changes in all role complexes over time, i.e., the lifespan of the family

Figure 5–1. Levels of abstraction of basic concepts of family developmental model.

(Bates, 1956; Deutscher, 1959; Farber, 1956) and represent different levels of abstraction (Hill & Rodgers, 1964). Note that by the definitions, as the concepts become more abstract they reflect the increasing importance of change over time. For example, *norm* represents a more or less static entity, an expectation for behavior, whereas *role sequence* or *career* cannot be defined without reference to the dimension of time. These terms imply that role changes occur over the history of the family. Moreover, the higher level concepts reflect more complex patterns of timing that exist within a family.

It is evident from these basic concepts that the family development framework generally focuses upon expected changes in family role structures and dynamics that occur over time with some degree of regularity (Aldous, 1978; Hill & Rodgers, 1964; Nock, 1982). Terkelsen (1980) also incorporates unexpected or "paranormative" changes, e.g., illness, birth of handicapped child, or divorce, into the framework. "Developmental task" is a concept borrowed from Erikson (1963) and Havinghurst (1977) and is used in this framework to make operational the opportunities for change that occur in the career of an individual or family (Duvall, 1971). Chronological time is not used to explain or predict change in the family. Rather, "family time" is marked off by the developmental issues or tasks which emerge in a sequential pattern and effect significant change in the family as a whole.

These developmental tasks are organized, on a broader level, in terms of developmental phases or stages. The designation of these developmental phases varies among the family development theorists, although the differences are minor. Duvall (1971) uses age-related expectations of the oldest child as the criterion for identifying her nine stages of family development. Duvall's stages have been revised into five stages by Solomon (1973). Rodgers (1962) formulated 24 stages, including developmental events of the youngest as well as the oldest child. In addition, Rodgers (1973) prefers the word "category" to "stages," to convey a continuity and flexibility across the family life-span. Others have included the status of the breadwinner, number of positions in the family, premarital life, and postparental and non-parental experiences in formulation of stages (Carter & McGoldrick, 1980; Minuchin, 1974; Terkelsen, 1980). Generally, developmental phases will follow the pattern of expansion–stability–contraction over the family career. Each phase represents a time of major role change within the family.

With each new phase, certain roles and developmental tasks become more and less salient. Duvall (1971) outlines individual and family developmental tasks that accompany each stage of family development. There is, however, a core of tasks that exists throughout most of the family lifespan: reproduction, physical maintenance, security and protection, education and socialization, status-conferring, recreation, and affection-giving (Hill & Rodgers, 1964). Similarly, Terkelsen (1980) identifies "survival" needs as well as developmental tasks as basic to family life. These and other tasks operate as an interface between the family system and its environment. The developmental task, then, is a concept that links the influences of individual family members upon the family to requirements and influences upon the family from the surrounding environment (Aldous, 1978; Hill & Rodgers, 1964).

Family

The family is defined as a "semi-closed system of interacting personalities which is composed of interrelated positions and roles defined by society" (Rodgers, 1964, p. 264) and is a unique and essential part of society. Moreover, this system is characterized by progressive change and transformation (Hill & Mattessich, 1979). Nock (1982) explains that the purpose of the phrase "semi-closed" is to distinguish the family as interdependent with rather than dependent upon the environment. In general, the family is viewed from three levels of analyses (Rodgers, 1973): 1) societal–transactional which addresses the transactions between family and other groups, and the function of the family in society as a major social system; 2) group–interactional which focuses upon the interrelationships of the members' roles and positions, group norms, group structure, and processes of interaction, and 3) individual–actional which emphasizes the influence of the individual member's developmental needs and values upon the family unit. For example, biological, perceptual, intellectual and other characteristics act to influence the congruence or disparity between family role expectations and role behavior of the individual.

The family unit is addressed primarily from the perspective of the uniqueness of each individual member (Hill & Hansen, 1960; Rowe, 1966). Developmental tasks, behavioral expectations, and maturational levels of the parents and children are considered to be the major sources of developmental change. A major issue in family development models is the "dovetailing" of individual and family developmental tasks (Aldous, 1978), the conflicting and complementary relationships that exist among these tasks. For example, family conflicts frequently arise out of the interaction between the mid-adulthood parent and the adolescent child who have developed opposing perspectives about life and death, sense of futurity, and personal goals (for a further examination of these differences, see Prosen, Toews, & Martin, 1981).

In summary, then, family developmentalists attribute the greatest degree of importance to the individual family members rather than to the family as a nuclear unit with children, and least importance to the family environment. All three facets, however, are considered essential to family development.

Family Environment

The environment is a critical element, although not a central focus, in the family development framework. By definition, development is a process of progressive change that occurs by interaction between a living system and its environment (Harris, 1957). The family environment is composed of some of the raw materials taken in by the family to promote functioning. These include the historical time in which the family is living; societal norms and role expectations for the family as a whole and each member; and goods and information used in such family functions as physical maintenance, protection, education, socialization, and recreation. In general, environmental influences are regarded as mediators of family development; the impetus for change originates within the family, with the environment acting secondarily to shape the outcome of the changes. External factors, then, are necessary but not sufficient of and by themselves to cause great movement in family development (Hill & Mattessich, 1979).

Family Health

A description of family health can be derived from the family development framework as a synchronization of positional careers. This synchrony is largely dependent upon the ability of each family member to meet his or her own growth responsibilities (Aldous, 1978) or developmental tasks as they emerge over the lifespan. Although, in one sense, the family is viewed as a context for continued individual development, so too is the individual a vehicle for the family's development.

The developmental progress of each member contributes to the overall development of the family, its ability to achieve group tasks, and enhances its repertoire of skills needed for productive transactions between family and society. Family health is assumed to be present when the family as a unit is able to perform its vital functions: 1) physical maintenance of members; 2) socialization into roles of family and other groups; 3) maintenance of members' motivation and sense of meaning; 4) maintenance of organization within the family and in family–environment interactions; and 5) the addition of members and release of mature members (Aldous, 1978; Duvall, 1971; Rodgers, 1973).

Family health is inextricably related to family developmental processes. Health behaviors can be made operational in terms of the achievement of developmental tasks and the processes involved in such achievements. For example, what interdependencies exist between members' developmental tasks? Is the timing of the emergence of a member's given task congruent with the overall family time and with societal time clocks? Do the developmental strivings of one member facilitate those of another and of the family as a whole? Health, then, like development, is not a linear or additive process. It is not merely the accumulation of developmental tools. Neither can it be said that a family with four developmentally capable members is twice as healthy as a family with two such members. Rather, family health implies a sense of organization, timing, meaning, and direction in the accomplishment of developmental tasks.

Family Health Problems

Problems in family health arise when there is a failure to integrate new norms and role expectations that arise at some point in the career of a member's position (Rodgers, 1962). This failure contributes not only to difficulties in individual and family functioning but also to future difficulties in incorporating other norms and role behaviors that normally occur over the lifespan. The birth of the family's first child is an example of a critical time for the integration of new norms and roles.

One method of classifying potential family health problems is according to the basic concepts of the developmental framework whereby one category includes those problems related to the *structural* concepts of the family, i.e., norm, role, position, role complex; and the second category refers to those problems concerning the *temporal* concepts, i.e., role sequence, positional career, family career (Hill & Rodgers, 1964). For example, an excess of family structure, such as too many positions, may exceed the family's ability to support individual developmental progress. This may be the case when triplets are born or when extended family members move in with the family. Alternatively, if a family member is absent, there may be a deficit in the number of positions needed to absorb vital family roles. A role cluster, e.g., "housewife," may be too large or not challenging enough for a family member. A family may face a critical event for which there is no norm to guide actions. In reference to the second category of problems, i.e., temporally related problems, dysynchronies can exist between the positional careers of two or more members. Roles may occur out of sequence (e.g., mandatory early retirement) or too close together (e.g., new parental and career responsibilities) and present potential problems.

Finally, from a broader perspective, family health can be described in terms of the ability of environmental elements to nurture family development. Governmental services, political and economic trends, social attitudes and agencies, etc., all can influence family functioning. And all, in turn, can prosper from the effects of healthy, developing families.

Although the family development framework offers rich ideas on requisites for family health, it has not yet evolved into a family therapy model. The therapist's role based on this framework is receiving increased attention. A nurse–therapist's approach to family therapy based upon a reformulation of this framework is described later.

ROGERS' NURSING MODEL AND REFORMULATIONS

Rogers (1970, 1980) describes human development in terms of three principles of development which are reflected within the family development framework. Rogers postulates that human development occurs in accordance with the homeodynamic principles of helicy, resonancy, and complementarity (later termed integrality). The principle of helicy describes development as an irreversible, purposeful, and innovative process that becomes increasingly complex. This increasing complexity is not chaotic but is characterized by a unique patterning and organization of each human system, i.e., resonancy. The principle of complementarity emphasizes the significance of interactions between person and environment in effecting developmental change. Development occurs within a non-linear four-dimensionality which Rogers (1980) describes as a relative present, extending out infinitely and encompassing past and future possibilities.

The family developmentalists' use of the term *family career* (Rodgers, 1973) in contrast to *family life cycle* is consistent with nursing's view of development as a unidirectional, irreversible process. The expansion–stability–contraction pattern of the family lifespan and the continual waxing and waning of various roles and family tasks resemble the rhythmic patterning of the individual's lifespan described in Rogers' (1980) resonancy principle. In addition, the idea of increasing complexity in development is evident in the family tasks which, early on, are relatively basic and become more complex as the family develops.

Developmental change as described by Aldous (1978) is consistent with the non-linear, non-mechanistic portrayal of development by Rogers (1970): change in the family system as a whole does not result from a series of stimulus–response relationships from member to member in a rippling effect. Rather, family change is postulated to occur among all members simultaneously when certain role changes or developmental strivings of one or more members reach a threshold of enough magnitude to effect a total change in the family. Families change through "creative leaps" after realizing a certain degree of confusion and disequilibrium (Hoffman, 1980). Dysfunctional patterns are then traded for new, more productive patterns.

The family development framework also purports a non-linear perspective of time. The concepts of historical time, social time, family time, and individual time are used to momentarily capture the multi-dimensionality of family development. Family development cannot be understood without awareness of its embeddedness in a particular historical period and within a particular societal time clock for developmental progression. A linear or chronological view of time has not been found useful in developmental models. Within one phase of development are vestiges of past developmental choices and the precursors of future roles. This is evident, for example, in the family of childrearing stage whose current life situation is affected by future expectations of the child's college education and the parents' retirement. "Each stage has its beginnings in the phases that are past and its fruition in development yet to come" (Duvall, 1971, p. 118). This implies an organization that is continually increasing in complexity and is directed toward a goal, i.e., fruition. Figure 5–2 outlines this multi-dimensionality of family development.

The two main axes (A and B) represent time dimensions of the family as a whole (axis A) and of the individual members (axes B). The multiple B axes identify each family member's unique set of development issues. Arrows on each axis indicate ongoing and irreversible change in family and positional careers. By definition, the term *career* implies this continual patterning over time (Aldous, 1978). The arrows belie the nonlinear and probablistic nature of the entire process; no one specific event can be iden-

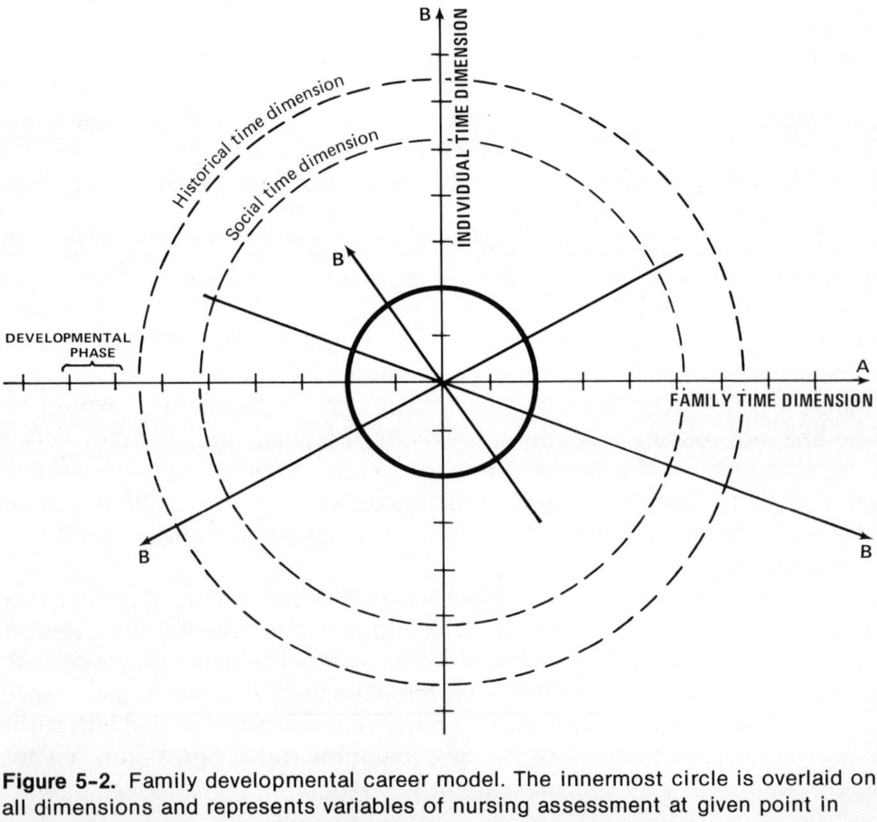

Figure 5–2. Family developmental career model. The innermost circle is overlaid on all dimensions and represents variables of nursing assessment at given point in space-time. **A** axis = family career. **B** axes = positional careers.

tified as the cause of family developmental change. The family developmental process is embedded in historical and social time dimensions (the two outermost circles) that influence those issues which become relevant. The innermost circle marks the point in space–time at which the nurse engages with the family. This point is described in terms of the developmental phase or transition the family is currently experiencing. This innermost circle is overlaid on all time dimensions; these are included to varying degrees in the nursing assessment of the family, i.e., historical, social, family, and individual time dimensions.

Family

Descriptions of the family within the family development framework are not entirely consistent with Rogers' (1970) open-system view of unitary man. The semi-closed nature of the family system needs to be modified to account for the openness of all living systems. This modification would then necessitate some reformulation concerning families' selective boundary maintenance behaviors. Less attention would be given to how the family maintains its boundary and more attention to ways in which the family integrates environmental influences and effects change in the environment, and to patterns of family–environment interaction that promote family health and development.

The definition of the family as a unity of interacting personalities does not necessarily conflict with a nursing perspective of human systems. Although there is a focus on the individuals within the family system in terms of their role positions, role sequences, etc., the developmental framework refrains from proposing an additive approach to interpreting the behavior of the family as a whole unit; family functioning is based upon more than the summation of each member's behavior (Carter & McGoldrick, 1980). However, except for the delineation of developmental tasks of the family as a whole, the developmental framework does not emphasize the family as a unit. Focus is directed instead toward individuals and subsystems, e.g., paired interactions, reciprocal roles, as they relate to the family. A reformulated model would build upon and emphasize developmental tasks of the family as a whole.

Family–Environment Interaction

Rogers' (1980) principle of complementarity describes the interaction between person and environment as an ongoing, mutual process. Family developmental tasks are understood to be manifestations of family–environment interaction (Hill & Rodgers, 1964). Figure 5–3 is an enlargement of a slice from the Family Developmental Career Model (Fig. 5–2) of family behavior and highlights the interaction between family and its environment. Note that the words *developmental strivings* can be used instead of the term *tasks* to emphasize the continuousness and goal-

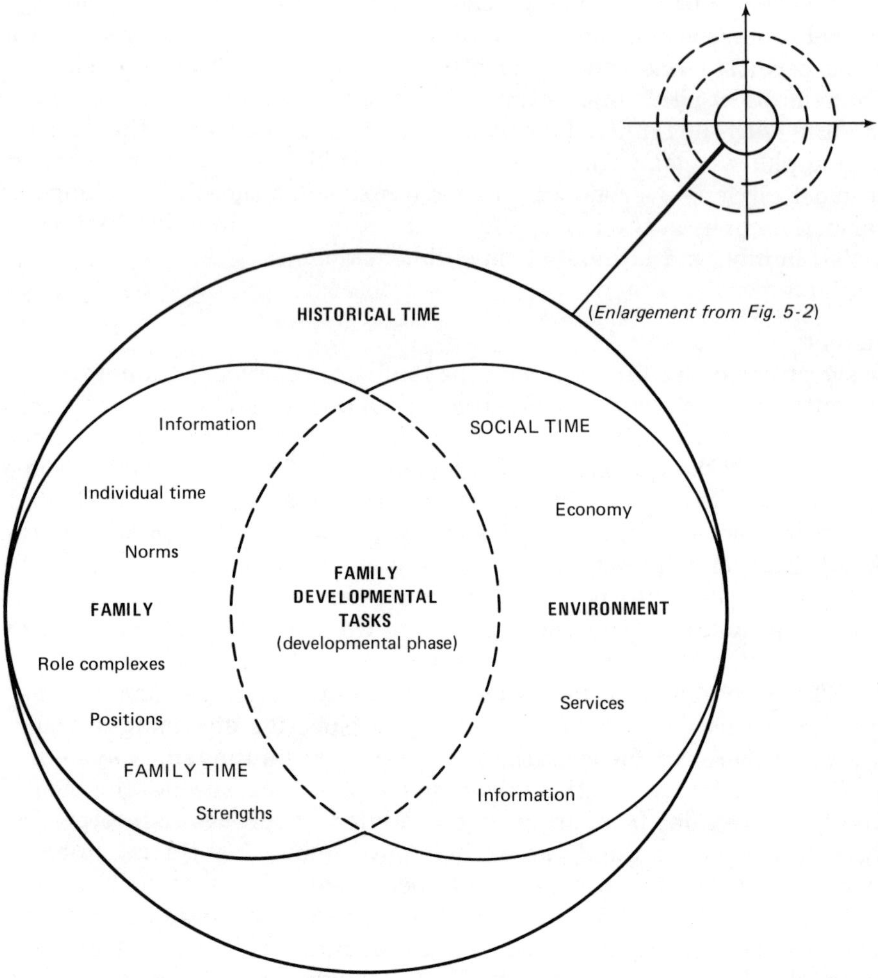

Figure 5-3. Family-environment interaction: developmental tasks.

directedness of the family's interaction with the environment (Nock, 1982).

Developmental tasks arise out of societal norms, individual maturational factors, and family needs and goals. Duvall's (1971) family task, "Facing the possibility of children and planning for their coming" (pp. 182–184) is an example of these multiple and mutual influences upon the family. The task is the outcome of a number of factors including social pressure, personal desire and need, and level of maturity. Achieving the task will bring the family into greater interactions with the environment in the form of material goods, community services, health care information, and financial counseling. Thus, one of the predominant concepts of the family development framework, developmental tasks, reflects a major nursing principle, i.e., complementarity. In addition, other basic concepts used to describe family behavior such as norm and role are based upon the assumption that family and society are interdependent.

Beyond this, however, there is some need for reformulation. The framework posits that the family is selectively open to the environment (Hill & Rodgers, 1964; Rodgers, 1973), contrary to Rogers' (1980) emphasis upon the complete, "not a little bit," openness of the human system (p. 331). Nock (1982) explains that this semi-openness implies a meaningful distinction between the family and its environment. Although Rogers (1970) identifies person and environment as two separate fields and agrees that there is pragmatic value for identifying boundaries around infinite energy fields, there is the basic assumption that human and environmental fields are in continuous interaction.

In the reformulation, the selectivity idea in the family framework could be salvaged and used instead to describe a selectivity regarding the *content* of interaction between family and environment. The ongoing and open *process* of interaction is inevitable. However, the family can make purposeful, intelligent choices or selections about the means of interaction. For example, the family can be viewed as interacting with society through choosing norms, values, peer groups, church organizations, methods of education, types of recreation, living arrangements, etc. This reformulation, then, achieves a consistency with the nursing perspective and enhances understanding of family potential for health and development.

Family Health

Health is a phenomenon of developmental processes in both Rogers' (1970, 1980) nursing conceptual model and the family development framework (Aldous, 1978; Duvall, 1971; Hill & Rodgers, 1964). Health is a manifestation of holistic, not additive, properties. The multiplicity of factors of each member, e.g., historical time, maturation, society, etc., that come together to influence synchrony in positional careers over the family lifespan cannot be examined separately and added together to predict health outcomes. Health is influenced by these factors, their interrelationships, and by unknown elements; the health process is more than a sum of the parts. Marital satisfaction, for example, cannot be determined by counting the number of husband/wife interactions or adding developmental accomplishments. Development is an emergent not reductionistic process (Hill & Mattessich, 1979). In this way, family health, as derived from the family developmental model, is consistent with the nursing perspective.

The major reformulation needed regarding what may be called family health behaviors in the framework is in reference to the approaches to change. The family is depicted as changing and developing generally by two approaches: adaptation and initiation (Aldous, 1978). This idea originates from the framework's assumption that the person is both actor and reactor. From a nursing perspective, however, the focus on "family adaptability to change" (Aldous, 1978, p. 35) would be shifted over to a more exclusive focus on health as a function of the family's ability to initiate change. This reformulation is guided by Rogers' (1970) description of human beings as goal-directed, purposeful, and innovative. Nursing assessment and interventions, then, would account for the family's potential and the skills for initiating needed changes.

In summary, nursing reformulations of the family development framework emphasize ongoing and innovative change within the family. Family change occurs out of interactions among members and between family and the broader environment. Developmental tasks are regarded as manifestations of these interactions. The increasing complexity of developmental tasks is balanced by an organization or a patterning that is characteristic of a family career. Individual, family, social, and historical time dimensions all influence the career of the family. Ultimately, family health is effected by purposeful choices initiated by the family about the ways in which the family will interact with the environment and pattern its developmental changes.

NURSE–THERAPISTS' APPROACH

The reformulated family development conceptual framework has significant implications for practitioners. The framework can be applied to promoting health in the family who follows expected developmental patterns and, also, in the family who deviates from the expected progression and may instead be expressing its own unique developmental patterning. The following paragraphs outline a nurse–therapist's approach to the assessment, diagnosis, intervention, and evaluation of family development problems.

Assessment

A primary focus for assessment within a reformulated developmental framework is the family time-dimensions:

1. What developmental phase or issues is the family presently experiencing?
2. What are the family tasks associated with that phase?
3. What is the three-generation profile of the family in terms of dates of birth, deaths, illnesses, separations, divorces, relocations, marriages, and retirement? (Hill, 1970). What is the profile of the family's normal pattern of major life changes over time?
4. What are the family's expectations for future patterning? Does the family indeed perceive a pattern to their life changes?

5. To what degree is the family's present experience synchronous with the overall family career?
6. How does the interaction between family and societal and historical time-dimensions affect family health?

The individual time-dimension is also important and is assessed in reference to data on family time:

1. What developmental phase or issues are salient for each family member?
2. What are the developmental tasks associated with that phase?
3. What is each member's positional career?
4. To what degree is the individual's developmental strivings synchronous with his or her past positional career?
5. How are past and future developmental issues manifested in the individual's present experiences?
6. To what degree is the individual's developmental strivings synchronous with the family career at the time of assessment? How many positional careers (i.e., size of family) exist in the family? What is their relatedness? Are they sufficient for family health?

This assessment outline reflects the significance of temporal variations and patterns inherent in family life. The developmental framework directs the practitioner more to an assessment of the timing of events and less to the content of the events (Aldous, 1978; Hill & Mattessich, 1979; Neugarten, 1979; Rodgers, 1973). A relevant question, for example, might be how a family involved in the launching phase facilitates the needs for an adult child still living at home. How, in this case, does the child's individual time clock conflict with the family time clock? What role might historical time have in this dysynchrony, (e.g., economic depression, early retirement of parent)? Does the social time clock dictate that it is inappropriate for the child to remain home? Attention to these dimensions of time—individual, family, social, and historical—is supported in part by Rogers' (1980) idea of four-dimensionality. They outline relevant domains for a developmental approach to family assessment. In addition, assessment must focus on patterns of interactions and events rather than isolated incidents (Alpert, 1981; Terkelsen, 1980). Events and interactions become meaningful only as they represent a patterning within a family.

This focus of assessment also allows for individual and family uniqueness and provides some flexibility in determining what is healthy development for a given family. In other words, the normality of a particular developmental experience is determined to a large degree by that family's developmental patterning and current perspectives and goals. The nursing approach to defining health incorporates the client's own values and perspectives on well-being.

Assessment may include other variables which affect the timing and achievement of developmental tasks. Aldous (1978) identifies three family patterns, i.e., communication, power, and affection, which influence family development. These patterns are evident through interactions between family members and change during the career of the family. Thus, internal as well as external and interactional factors are a part of the family assessment.

In addition, it is important to maintain awareness that family developmental patterning is a non-linear process in that it is likely to be unrelated to chronological time (age). Lifespan developmental frameworks attribute little value to this linear measurement of change. Instead, interactions within the family and between the family and environment are likely to have a much stronger relationship to developmental progression.

Diagnosis

Rogers (1970, p. 127) gives direction to the types of diagnoses that emerge from a holistic, developmental framework:

> Nursing diagnosis encompasses the man–environment relationship and seeks to identify sequential, cross-sectional patterning in the life process.

Given this and the developmental framework, nursing diagnoses of the family would identify problems and potential problems related to developmental tasks and their sequencing among family members. Some examples are:

1. Lack of integration of adolescent needs for independence into family system
2. Conflicts related to unemployed, middle-age parent and maintenance of family morale
3. Difficulty in "releasing" deceased (or divorced) family member by family in school-age stage of development
4. Decreased marital satisfaction related to problems in developing relationships with in-laws during the establishment phase
5. Inability to resolve conflict between parental career/occupational tasks and family maintenance needs within family of childbearing stage

These examples indicate how the timing of personal developmental events (adolescence, middle-age, death, marriage), historical time (economic unemployment, dual-parent employment), social norms ("parents are breadwinners," "death is inappropriate before retirement phase of life," "parents are the primary caregivers during the childrearing stage") and stage of family development can result in family problems. The conflicts arise from the convergence of developmental issues at a certain point in time. As individual, family, societal, and historical development occurs and the developmental variables are rearranged, old problems may abate and new ones emerge. Thus, any listing of nursing diagnoses of "typical" family problems would require ongoing review and possible revision.

Intervention

Nursing intervention with families is directed toward promoting "rhythmic consistencies" (Rogers, 1970, p. 23) or "good life-cycle management" (Hill, 1970, p. 323); that is, promoting a synchronization of the changes that occur across positional careers in a family. This synchrony does not imply that all members must share the same developmental concerns at the same time, nor does it imply that conflict is unhealthy. Rather, "synchrony" defines a family experience wherein various developmental strivings occurring simultaneously come together in a way that produces positive *patterning* of family functioning. Think, for example, of an elaborate array of dominoes, each standing on end beside one another. The position and motion of each domino as it falls is different but, if each domino is positioned correctly, the timing of each domino's fall will produce a coherent pattern that can be observed.

Interventions, then, would include helping the family in decision making about the timing and positional careers related to certain developmental events such as marriage, childbearing, education, career, and retirement. Parents, for example, may be guided in purposefully timing changes in career, residence, or financial status so as to complement the emotional, social, and educational needs of young family members and contribute to overall family harmony. These events represent times when there may be significant role choices and changes that would ultimately affect the health and well-being of family members.

Knowledge of developmental needs of individuals and families can be translated to family members in a way that assists them in anticipating critical periods, e.g., sibling rivalry or bereavement, and in providing a family environment that facilitates the development of children and parents. The family can also be helped to perceive the normality in the developmental strivings of its members and potential conflicts. Problems can occur when a family impedes the developmental process of change by attempting to ignore conflict and maintain the status quo. Family health, from a developmental view, thrives on a certain degree of disequilibrium and ongoing change. Thus, the therapist would work toward maintaining "developmental momentum" (Terkelsen, 1980) by first acknowledging the normality of and need for the developmentally based conflict.

These interventions occur ideally before major problems surface. High-risk families could be identified as recipients of these interventions, the goal being that such information would reduce the probability of future family problems. Low-risk families as well as families who are already experiencing difficulties can also benefit from these health-promotive interventions.

Family problems that do arise represent opportunities (and need) for further development. The therapeutic goal is to restore developmental momentum (Terkelsen, 1980) or "remobilize" the family (Haley, 1973). The disorganization and ambiguity of family conflicts are fertile ground for the emergence of new, more useful role behaviors, perspectives, and patterns of interaction among family members, i.e., patterns that propel the family into the next developmental stage. The nurse first helps the family identify the developmental tasks at hand, the previous attempts at achieving them, the ways in which they may impinge upon others, and the resources acquired from previously achieved tasks (Critchley, 1982). Goals are set regarding productive ways to achieve individual and family tasks. The family, stimulated by the exigencies of the current situation, is then allowed and encouraged to improvise or innovate roles and positions and to test out the new family patterns that result. (Also see Hughes, Berger, & Wright, 1978; Weeks & Wright, 1979, for clinical illustrations of facilitating family developmental change.)

This intervention approach taps into the family's (like all living systems') developmental potential to create order out of chaos, i.e., negentropy. Aldous (1978, p. 59) explains that people's behaviors "are increasingly the result of improvisation rather than that of rigidly prescribed norms." Family members possess role-*making* as well as role-*taking* abilities. The potential for pro-active rather than re-active family behaviors is highlighted by the nurse–therapist.

The nurse can facilitate purposeful behaviors in times of family career dysynchrony. Families can be assisted to "compensate for timing failures" (Aldous, 1978, p. 334). The family who has reared a poorly socialized child can be taught healthier parent–child interaction patterns and ways to enrich the family environment so as to promote development that has not yet occurred. In addition, particular deficits in child or parents can be identified and addressed in therapy to facilitate other developmental goals.

Evaluation

Intervention outcomes would be evaluated in reference to particular therapy goals, the family's ability to carry out family functions, and the family's ability to promote a sense of direction and accomplishment in current developmental strivings. Questions similar to those outlined in the assessment would be asked with the expectation that the family is better able to identify its tasks, to perceive developmental patterns in its history of family experiences, and to engage in behaviors that promote synchrony in the family career.

Case Example

Lisa is a 13-year-old who has run away from home for the second time. She is described as an intelligent girl, but a loner. She is the youngest of four children and was born, as her parents readily admit, from an unplanned, unwanted pregnancy. Her older siblings are grown and have left home.

Lisa's mother, age 47, recently received a promotion at her job, which she has found to be a meaningful distraction from Lisa's ongoing behavior problems. Lisa's father, age 49, is looking forward to early retirement and moving to a warm climate. He is proud of the accomplishments of his three older sons and once held high expectations for Lisa. More recently, his goal is "to get Lisa graduated and out on her own."

Lisa's family presented themselves at the family mental health clinic for help soon after police returned Lisa to her home. The nurse's family intervention began with a positive comment noting that all three members of the family had come. The family was introduced to the philosophy and general goals of therapy and their perspectives about the problem were explored. Major areas of assessment of this family included Lisa's past developmental achievements and current strivings, as well as those of each of her parents. Periods of potential conflict between members and their developmental tasks were noted and validated with the family. Lisa's current problem-causing behaviors were assessed in reference to previous patterns of interacting with her parents, teachers, and classmates. Lisa's brothers were invited to join the sessions but refused, stating that they would not be able to help.

Lifespan developmental concepts were used by the nurse as a guide in identifying normal or expected behaviors across each member's lifespan. The family's own unique developmental pattern was also used in formulating a profile of their family career. Lisa's birth initiated a second phase of childbearing/childrearing/child-launching for the family whereas family members had patterned their lives more after the first childbearing phase which included her three older brothers. Lisa's own career in the family generated conflicts with the family's overall expectations and intensified the disparity between the mother's and father's individual goals. A diagnosis was formulated: family conflict between parental expectations and role behaviors of an adolescent daughter.

Interventions were based upon the dysynchronies that had unfolded from interactions between the positional careers of Lisa's mother and father, and Lisa. The family was helped to understand how the timing of Lisa's birth may have been incompatible with the parents' developmental stages and how this experience initiated a pattern of interaction that conveyed some resentment and rejection toward her. Their present problems were regarded as an expression of the family's history as well as their present.

The timing of the mother's promotion at work and her developmental needs to be productive were presented in reference to Lisa and her negative expressions of continuing needs for nurturance and self-esteem. Similarly, the nurse elicited the family's views about the father's movement along his career which seemed out of step with Lisa's current developmental needs; his anticipation of a "contraction" of the family career conflicted with Lisa's need for a sense of family stability and security as she began to wrestle with independence–dependence issues of adolescence. The dysynchrony between the two parents' developmental tasks of middle-age were also explored in sessions with and without Lisa, employing their differing career patterns as a springboard for discussion of other, more personal developmental concerns and the ways in which Lisa may have intensified their impact.

The parents were helped to restructure their perceptions about age-related expectations for Lisa. They came to realize that Lisa's developmental career was different from that of her older, now grown-up brothers. Lisa's school and family environment were different and her interactions within these unique situations influenced developmental patterns that differed from her older siblings.

Approaches to enriching the family environment were identified that would facilitate all members' developmental strivings. The father reconsidered his timing for retirement and the mother reevaluated her motives for focusing so intently upon her job. Lisa learned more about her own needs and those of her parents. The normality of the developmental tasks were emphasized by the nurse, as was the family's potential to establish a functional pattern of positional careers among themselves. The family was encouraged to create a source of family enjoyment and to include it in their regular family schedule.

The movement toward healthier family patterns was not easy for Lisa and her family. Members worked to enhance their position in the family by giving up some non-productive roles and developing new roles and patterns of interaction. Lisa learned other, more communicative ways to express feelings of conflict with her family. This was particularly crucial for Lisa because she was perched on the edge of a developmental phase which normally brings increased family tension. As her needs for intimacy and self-confidence were beginning to be met through her family, she was able to take risks in extending trust in herself and her family out toward a trust in others. She became increasingly able to engage in genuine relationships with peers and teachers. Thus, the problem which brought the family into therapy was alleviated or, more accurately, transformed into more productive family behaviors. The path of the family career prior to therapy had found a new direction for development.

SIGNIFICANCE AND FUTURE DIRECTIONS

The family development framework is a conceptual model which, with nursing reformulations, has implications for nursing intervention in promoting family well-being. The reformulated model lacks clear measures of achievement of tasks and has not yet attained strong empirical support for identification of the various family phases (Alpert & Richardson, 1980; Nock, 1982). In view of the lack of such a taxonomy, it is suggested that identification of potential or actual problems in family development be based upon an assessment of developmental events of individual members which contribute to marked changes in positional careers within the family. The following developmental events have the potential of altering family positional careers and roles: birth, death, a child's progression through school, job change, unemployment, child's graduation or marriage, divorce, remarriage, and retirement. These and other events are integral to family development and are due largely to the complex historical and social time dimensions in which today's families exist: a child's marriage or graduation does not necessarily mark a postparental phase for the parents; childbearing may occur in the second or even third decade of marriage; a family may experience several job careers throughout its lifespan; the point at which children enter school is blurred by day-care and preschool options that are becoming the norm; and older adulthood is not necessarily accompanied by grandchildren or retirement. Thus, broad categories of family stages outlined by Duvall (1971), Aldous (1978), and others may not be sensitive enough to alert the nurse to critical developmental issues occurring within a particular family.

Clearly, there is a need for research into the significance and usefulness of the reformulated family development framework. Research of an exploratory nature could focus on surveying family therapy records for problems and diagnoses that represent developmental issues. The question could then be explored as to whether the developmental tasks of certain family members have greater or lesser influence upon the overall family developmental progress. For example, does achievement of tasks in the expectant father, e.g., identification with the parental role, relate to family adjustment after the birth of the baby? There is need for research into the potentially significant relationships between individual members' developmental tasks and developmental tasks of the family as a whole.

Another area of research is in reference to universal family developmental tasks. Is there a core of developmental issues that are significant to family health across families of the same culture? Of different cultures? (See Komagai, 1984). Some authors propose a universal set of tasks (Barcai, 1981) while others are critical of this idea (Wright & Leahey, 1984). Moreover, the same developmental task, e.g., parental job change, could be studied longitudinally within families for its influence upon family health at different points in time. The same developmental event may promote family development at one time yet inhibit it at another.

Significant research based on a family developmental model cannot overlook the need for an empirically based taxonomy of family stages. An inductive approach to research could contribute to building knowledge about the existence of these stages and the tasks associated with each stage. Specific tasks might then function to make operative and measure the level of attainment of a particular family developmental stage. Differences and commonalities in family developmental stages could be clarified across a variety of family situations, e.g., first marriage, single-parent, and remarriage (Whiteside, 1982).

Approaches to research could address questions designed to test Rogers' (1980) principles of helicy, resonancy, or complementarity and their applicability to understanding family functioning:

1. Do family developmental tasks display an increase in complexity and organization over the career of a family? In what ways are these characteristics manifested? (Helicy)
2. What developmental patternings exist within and across families? How do these patternings compare across families? (Resonancy)

3. What roles do societal and historical time dimensions have in family development? Are there times when certain dimensions play a more or less significant role in the family? (Complementarity)

Eventually, interventions that incorporate a developmental approach in family therapy will be derived from previous research findings and the emerging theory. These interventions could then be tested using a quasi-experimental research design. This research would measure the effectiveness of developmentally based family interventions as compared to more traditional modes of family therapy. The findings may provide evidence that would lend support to a family developmental therapy model.

In summary, the family development framework is still very much in the process of theory development. It is, however, currently regarded as a significant family conceptual model primarily because of its ability to handle the inevitable change that is experienced in families at various levels, i.e., individual members, family, and environment, and within different units of time (Hill, 1970; Hill & Mattessich, 1979; Rodgers, 1964). Jones and Dimond (1982) describe the developmental framework as a family theory model that transcends the static, closed-systems views of the structural–functional and interactional family theory models, and as a useful framework for practice.

The reformulated family development framework offers even greater possibilities for better understanding the family and the nurse–therapist's approach. It provides guidelines for predicting the "nature and direction of [the family's] development" (Rogers, 1970, p. 139) and may serve to make Rogers' developmental concepts available for use in practice. There is need for research to improve its theoretical structure and explanatory power for use in planning interventions and predicting outcomes. How do temporal variations in developmental tasks among family members give rise to healthy family patterns? Researchers are challenged to answer such questions. Practitioners are challenged to continue to purposefully address the developmental phenomena essential to the well-being of their families.

FOUR CENTRAL COMPONENTS OF NURSING APPROACHES

- **Title of Chapter:** The Developmental Conceptual Framework: Nursing Reformulations and Applications for Family Therapy
- **Definitions**

  Family: An open system of developing individuals, each of whom has a positional career that is interrelated with the family career.
- **Family Environment:** The historical and social time dimensions in which the family lives, and the goods and information taken in by the family to promote functioning.

- **Family Health:** A synchronization of positional careers.
- **Therapist's Role:** To facilitate family development by promoting synchronization of the changes that occur across positional careers. Interventions include but are not limited to: education for good life-cycle management; anticipatory guidance on developmental tasks; assisting in decision making on timing of positional career changes; and facilitating repatterning of members' developmental strivings by improving new patterns out of dysynchronous family patterns.

REFERENCES

Aldous, J. (1978). *Family careers: Developmental changes in families.* New York: Wiley.

Alpert, J. L. (1981). Theoretical perspective on the family life cycle. *Counseling Psychologist, 9* (4), 25–34.

Alpert, J. L., & Richardson, M. S. (1980). Parenting. In L. W. Poon (Ed.), *Aging in the 1980's.* Washington, D.C.: American Psychological Association. pp. 441–454.

Barcai, A. (1981). Normative family development. *Journal of Marital and Family Therapy, 7*(3), 353–359.

Bates, F. L. (1956). Position, role, and status: A reformulation of concepts. *Social Forces, 34,* 313–321.

Carter, E. A., & McGoldrick, M. (1980). The family life cycle and family therapy: An overview. In E. A. Carter & M. McGoldrick (Eds.), *The family life cycle: A framework for family therapy.* (pp. 3–20). New York: Gardner Press.

Critchley, D. L. (1982). A developmental perspective for treatment of families with young children. In T. W. Clements & D. M. Buchanan (Eds.), *Family therapy: A nursing perspective* (pp. 267–276). New York: Wiley.

Deutscher, I. (1959). *Married life in the middle years.* Kansas City: Community Studies.

Duvall, E. M. (1971). *Family development* (4th ed.). Philadelphia: Lippincott.

Erikson, E. H. (1963). *Childhood and society* (2nd ed.). New York: W. W. Norton & Co., Inc.

Farber, B. (1956). *A model for the study of the family as mutually contingent careers.* Ph.D. dissertation, University of Illinois.

Haley, J. (1973). *Uncommon therapy: The psychiatric techniques of Milton H. Erickson.* New York: W. W. Norton & Co., Inc.

Harris, D. B. (1957). Problems in formulating a scientific concept of development. In D. B. Harris (Ed.), *The concept of development* (pp. 3–14). Minneapolis: University of Minnesota Press.

Havinghurst, R. J. (1977). *Developmental tasks and education* (3rd ed.). New York: D. McKay.

Hill, R. (1970). *Family development in three generations.* Cambridge, Mass.: Schenkman.

Hill, R., & Hansen, D. A. (1960). The identification of conceptual frameworks utilized in family study. *Marriage and Family Living, 22,* 299–311.

Hill, R., & Mattessich, P. (1979). Family development theory and life-span development. In P. B. Baltes & O. G. Brim, Jr. (Eds.), *Life-span development and behavior (Vol. 2).* New York: Academic Press.

Hill, R. & Rodgers, R. H. (1964). The developmental approach. In H. T. Christensen (Ed.), *Handbook of marriage and the family* (pp. 171–214). Chicago: Rand McNally.

Hoffman, L. (1980). The family life cycle and discontinuous change. In E. A. Carter & M. McGoldrick (Eds.), *The family life cycle: A framework for family therapy* (pp. 53–68). New York: Gardner Press.

Hughes, S., Berger, M., & Wright, L. (1978). The family life cycle and clinical interventions. *Journals of Marriage and Family Counseling, 4,* 33–40.

Jones, S. L., & Dimond, M. (1982). Family theory and family therapy models: Comparative review with implications for nursing practice. *Journal of Psychosocial Nursing, 20* (10), 12–19.

Komagai, F. (1984). The life cycle of the Japanese family. *Journal of Marriage and the Family, 46,* (191–204).

Minuchin, S. (1974). *Families and family therapy.* Cambridge, Mass.: Harvard University Press.

Neugarten, B. L. (1979). Time, age and the life cycle. *American Journal of Psychiatry, 136*(7), 887–894.

Newman, M. (1979). *Theory development in nursing.* Philadelphia: F. A. Davis.

Nock, S. L. (1982). The life-cycle approach to family analysis. In B. B. Wolman (Ed.), *Handbook of Developmental Psychology* (pp. 636–651). Englewood Cliffs, N. J.: Prentice-Hall.

Parse, R. R. (1981). *Man-living-health: A theory of nursing.* New York: Wiley.

Prosen, H., Toews, J., & Martin, R. (1981). The life cycle of the family: Parental midlife crisis and adolescent rebellion. *Adolescent Psychiatry, 9,* 180–198.

Rodgers, R. H. (1962). *Improvements in the construction and analysis of family life cycle categories.* Ph.D. dissertation, Western Michigan University.

Rodgers, R. H. (1964). Toward a theory of family development. *Journal of Marriage and the Family, 26,* 262–270.

Rodgers, R. H. (1973). *Family interaction and transaction: The developmental approach.* Englewood Cliffs, N.J.: Prentice-Hall.

Rodgers, M. E. (1970). *An introduction to the theoretical basis of nursing.* Philadelphia: F.A. Davis.

Rogers, M. E. (1980). Nursing: A science of unitary man. In J. P. Riehl & C. Roy (Eds.), *Conceptual models for nursing practice* (pp. 329–338). New York: Appleton-Century-Crofts.

Rowe, G. P. (1966). The developmental conceptual framework to the study of the family. In F. I. Nye & F. M. Berardo (Eds.), *Emerging conceptual frameworks in family analysis* (pp. 198–222). New York: Macmillan.

Solomon, M. A. (1973). A developmental, conceptual premise for family therapy. *Family Process, 12,* 179–188.

Terkelsen, K. G. (1980). Toward a theory of the family life cycle. In E. A. Carter & M. McGoldrick (Eds.), *The family life cycle: A framework for family therapy* (pp. 3–20). New York: Gardner Press.

Weeks, G. R., & Wright, L. (1979). Dialectics of family life cycle. *American Journal of Family Therapy, 7,* 85–91.

Whiteside, M. F. (1982). Remarriage: A family developmental process. *Journal of Marital and Family Therapy, 8,* 59–68.

Wright, L. M., & Leahey, M. (1984). *Nurses and families: A guide to family assessment and intervention.* Philadelphia: F. A. Davis.

— APPROACH THREE

Use of an Inductively Derived Nursing Approach to Reformulate an Existing Family Therapy Theory

6

A Reformulation of the Interactional Approach to Family Therapy

Susan L. Jones

INTRODUCTION: THE FOUNDERS AND BEGINNING OF THE MODEL

One of the most prominent theoretical approaches to family therapy is the Interactional approach, developed in the 1950s and 1960s. This chapter examines the Interactional approach to family therapy in light of an inductively derived eclectic nursing model. Family therapy concepts of the Interactional model are first explained and then reformulated into a family nursing approach.

What is here termed the *Interactional* approach has been called elsewhere the "strategic" or the "communication" approach (Haley, 1976a; Foley, 1974). Similar to other family therapy approaches, this theoretical model was conceptualized out of research initially attempting to link schizophrenia and family dynamics. The important question was: "Are there specific family dynamics which cause schizophrenia in a child?" A family manifesting such dynamics was then referred to as "schizophrenogenic family."

Several people were involved in conceptualizing this model while working on two research projects: the Gregory Bateson (Double Bind) Project, and the Mental Research Institute, originally founded by Don D. Jackson. Because the two research endeavors are closely related, they have frequently been confused. Jackson, a primary contributor to the Interactional model, was associated with both projects. He worked as a consultant to the Bateson project during its existence from 1952 to 1962, and in 1958 he founded the Mental Research Institute (MRI). The Bateson project terminated in 1962 at which time two members of that project, Jay Haley and John Weakland, joined the staff of MRI. The fact that the two projects were housed in the same building for a period of time further contributed to the confusion between them (Jones, 1980).

Gregory Bateson began the Double Bind project in 1952; shortly after Jay Haley and John Weakland joined the staff. Don Jackson and William Fry became part-time consultants. The project lasted 10 years (Sluzki & Ransom, 1976; Berger, 1978). As its name indicates, the major thrust of the project was study of the double bind concept and its potential etiological relationship to schizophrenia. The double bind theoretical formulation consisted of a theory of communication in which dysfunctional communication patterns were considered to be a cause of schizophrenia (Bateson, et al., 1956). From the initial double bind concept, however, came a more general theory of communication in which dysfunctional communications were investigated generally within both sick and nonsymptomatic families (Sluzki & Ransom, 1976). The communication patterns were considered important, not only for their etiological role in the development of pathology, but also for their importance in a therapeutic relationship. Communication, therefore, is considered by the Bateson group as the foundation for the interactional approach to family therapy (Jones, 1980).

Midway through the double bind project, it was administratively divided into an experimental project and a family therapy (treatment) project. The experimental project examined double bind situations in detail and potential outcomes related to the double bind communications. Gradually, the research team became a treatment team in which the practice of family therapy was born. The family therapy that was conducted in those early days was termed *conjoint family therapy* and provided the basis for the strategies today known as Interactional techniques of family therapy.

One might say that the theory of communication at the Bateson Double Bind project expanded to a theory of interaction at the MRI project. Whereas communication provided the common denominator for research and therapy for the Bateson project, communication and behavior were considered to be synonymous for the MRI team (Greenberg, 1977). All behavior was considered to be communication so that interactional behaviors rather than words only became the unit of analysis. Major emphasis was placed on the interactional quality of the behaviors, that is, how the behaviors of one family member were shaped in relation to the behaviors of another family member.

Those theorists and therapists who founded the Interactional model of family therapy were very clear in their contention that this family therapy approach comprised a new theory of dysfunctional behavior and treatment for the behavior. It was not simply a compilation of new techniques based on previous psychiatric or psychological theories. Rather, it was a new way of analyzing human behavior and treating dysfunctional human behavior. They considered the approach unique because it stemmed from a new epistemological orientation which incorporated principles from cybernetics and general systems theory (Jones, 1980).

Examination of the Interactional model (as we shall see below) supports the contention that this paradigm is a new way of viewing human behavior and of intervening in dysfunctional behavior. Focus throughout the formulations has consistently been on the interactions between family members and the reciprocity of these interactions. Today there are several family therapy proponents of this paradigm, some of whom were involved in the original research of the Double Bind project or the MRI work. Others are more recent advocates. While the proponents such as Jackson, Haley, Weakland, Satir, and Watzlawick, et al differ in their respective points of view (both past and current), they all view a change in interactional patterns as the cornerstone of therapy.

THE UNIT OF TREATMENT

There are two ways by which one might consider the unit of treatment in family therapy. First is the locus of pathology for individual and family dysfunction, and second is delineation of who participates in the family therapy treatment. The first is an etiological issue and the second is a treatment issue.

Considering the etiological issue, the major starting point for these theorists was rejection of intradynamic concepts as the focus for causation. Instead, the unit of analysis involved the dynamics of interchange between individuals in the family; thus the name Interactional analysis developed (Jones, 1980). The assumption of such an approach is that individual pathology results from the way family members behave toward one another. That is, individual pathology results from interchanges in the family environment. All human problems result from interactional–situational difficulties (external social forces in the family environment) which can be identified at a particular point in time.

Because problem formation is caused by forces in the external family environment, problem alleviation results when the family social context is successfully manipulated. In this sense, the locus of pathology is seen as outside the individual and within the family environmental context.

Also important in this etiological theory of individual and family dysfunction is the contention of these theorists that they did not deny the existence of intrapsychic forces that influence human functioning. Their major shift from traditional psychiatric theories of human behavior at that time, however, was their argument that one cannot know the perceptions of another or the internal dynamics of another. Any therapy, to be successful, must operate on observable phenomena between individuals (Greenberg, 1977). The observable phenomena conceptualized as the treatment unit for these theorists was the interactional behaviors between family members.

The second manner by which we consider the unit of treatment in the Interactional family therapy approach is discussion of who participates in the family therapy sessions. In the early phases, Jackson and his associates believed that the entire family must be present during all therapy sessions (Jones, 1980). Subsequently, they decided that family interaction patterns could be modified by treating various family members without the entire family being there. Today, various combinations of individual family members attending the sessions over the course of therapy are used.

FAMILY HEALTH AND ILLNESS

Therapists of the Interactional approach view the family as a system of interactive behaviors (where all behavior is communication) (Jones, 1980). According to Jackson (1967), the family is an interlocking system where each member is a subsystem that influences all other members. Watzlawick (1967, 1974, 1977) discusses the family as a system of communication which is equivalent to a behavioral system. Again, communication is equated with behavior. Haley (1963) and Satir (1967a) support this definition, although Haley emphasizes the importance of power in any relationship while Satir emphasizes the importance of feelings.

A healthy functioning family is one in which the communications between individuals are clear. Each family member interacts with each other family member in a comfortable manner, that is, without the need to read into the other's behaviors or communication. The two family members understand the communications between them.

Each theorist of this approach outlines a healthy functioning family in a slightly different way. Development of conceptual theories that discussed Interactional units in a relationship allowed Jackson, Haley, Watzlawick, and Satir to move from intradynamic constructs to observable phenomena that could be made operational as behavioral communication between family members. Thus, a healthy functioning family could be described in behavioral (communication) terms.

Jackson developed the "Rules Hypothesis" or "Quid Pro Quo." In this hypothesis, he argued that family member *A*'s response to family member *B* was limited by *B*'s response to *A*. As a result, family members react to each other in repetitive ways because the range of responses is limited as shown by the following diagram. The repetition in the process of the interactions shows that certain rules (family rules) govern what sort of relationship can occur.

Such an hypothesis of family functioning makes sense when we consider that healthy family functioning occurs when the rules are clear and

Responses ruled by a quid pro quo

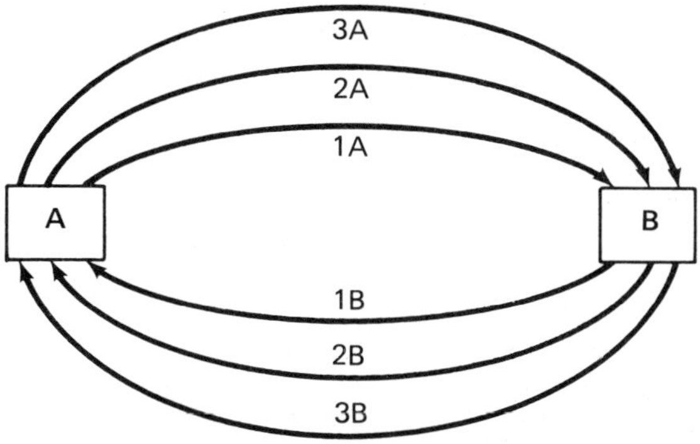

Where 1A is limited by 1B and 1B is limited by 1A;
2A is limited by 2B and 2B is limited by 2A, etc.

well formulated, and unhealthy family functioning occurs when the rules are unclear and not well formulated. Considering that the family is an organization, clear rules of operation are needed (Jackson, 1965a; 1965b; 1967). Following the rules hypothesis, all family activity, even if it seemed bizarre (dysfunctional) initially, would make sense (be functional) if the rules under which the behavior occurred were formulated.

Jackson (1965a; 1965b) and Haley (1959; 1963; 1971) both speculated on the manner by which the family rules adapted to change and particularly how they developed initially. The important contribution of Haley in explaining healthy and unhealthy family functioning is his discussion of *power* in family relationships. According to Haley, any two people who interact begin to work out what sort of behavior (communication) is to take place in that relationship. More important, however, is the fact that they are working out a higher level problem: who is to decide, or control, what sort of behavior is to take place (Jones, 1980). They work out the relationship in terms of power.

As the two persons interact, each message, by the fact of its existence, implies that it belongs in the relationship. Also, each message is qualified by other messages. Implicit in each qualifying message is the attempt to work out who is in control or who is to decide what type of messages and behavior is to take place in the relationship. In a healthy family relationship the deciding is shared. *A* offers *B* a message, *B* counters with one of his own, and each indicates that he is deciding what behavior is to take place and, therefore, what sort of relationship it is, as shown in the following diagram.

One example discussed is that of a couple who meet for the first time. In the beginning, a wide range of behaviors could occur. Over time, however, there is a selection of certain behaviors and the couple begins to negotiate agreements; they begin to establish rules about what each

Healthy family functioning

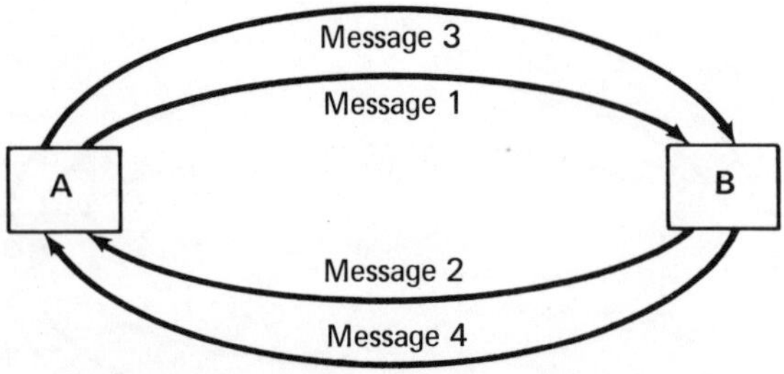

Where Message 2 takes into account Message 1;
Message 3 takes into account Message 2, etc., to formulate the relationship through *mutual* decision making.

can do and say. Similarly, they begin to negotiate the process by which such behaviors are decided upon. Such mutual exchanges represent the essence of the relationship and exemplify healthy family functioning.

Jackson (1965b; 1968) uses the concept of quid pro quo to describe a relationship that has well-formulated rules. Integral to the quid pro quo is the notion of the contract (the rule) and the process (the formula) by which it is developed. Jackson likens marriage to a legal contract in which each person receives something for which he must give something in return; a tit-for-tat sort of arrangement (Jones, 1980). No matter what tasks are pursued—making money, parenting, shopping, or whatever—the marital couple will arrive at an unwritten set of ground rules such that each person will behave in a certain manner in relation to the other person. When the unwritten ground rules are established, it is a quid pro quo arrangement. The more functional the relationship, the more clearly delineated are the ground rules in terms of contract and process by which they are formed.

Virginia Satir (1967b), in general, follows the thinking of Jackson when she considers the concept of family rules. Family rules are considered the mechanism by which family business gets done. Satir, however, incorporates the concept of values. Family rules express the value system by which the family operates and implies the concept of "should." The importance of the values is that they show how the family is influenced by the cultural context in which they live. In general, it is fair to say that dysfunctional families have dysfunctional rules since one begets the other. Frequently the family does not know what is happening, because they are unaware of the unwritten (and perhaps) dysfunctional rules by which they abide.

Watzlawick, like the theorists outlined above, emphasizes the repititious patterns (rules) operating in interactions between family members. When the rules are clear and the process of interactions is clear, the result is healthy family functioning. When there is not clarity in terms of contract or process, there is dysfunctional family functioning. In *Pragmatics of Human Communication*, Watzlawick and colleagues (1967) conceptualize the repetitious patterns of interactions through five axioms of communication. Because all behavior is communication, these five axioms define what type of interaction will occur in any relationship.

The first axiom states the impossibility of not communicating. No such thing exists as non-behavior; thus, one cannot not behave and one cannot not communicate. Whether the person is active or inactive, loud or silent, all behaviors have communication value and influence others—who in turn cannot not respond to these communications and are in themselves communicating in the process.

The second axiom states that all communication implies a commitment and defines a relationship. Not only is information conveyed in the communication process, but also the interaction imposes behavior.

The third axiom states that the nature of a relationship is contingent upon the punctuation sequence. Following Bateson, Jackson (1963; 1966) described punctuation as occurring when two persons in communication impose some type of order and causal sequence to the communication. An example of an Interactional sequence in the family of a chronically alcoholic husband is given by Greenberg (1977, p. 399):

> The husband would relate: my wife nags me; therefore, I withdraw and drink. The wife notes: he drinks and comes home disoriented and filthy, so I get after him to get his act together. Was it the wife who precipitated the withdrawal or the husband who initiated the nagging?

The fourth axiom is closely related to the second and states that human beings communicate both verbally (digitally) and non-verbally (analogically). The former allows for adequate communication on a content level but does not tell us much about the emotional level of a relationship. The latter tells us about the emotional aspects of the relationship but not all. Tears can be of sorrow or joy, a smile may be a sign of acceptance or contemptuous rejection.

Fifth is the axiom of symmetrical and complementary interactions, that is, all communicational exchanges are either symmetrical or complementary, based upon the kind of relationship that exists. If equality exists and either party is free to take the lead, a symmetrical relationship exists. If one leads and the other follows, a complementary relationship exists. Each term is meant to be descriptive rather than evaluative and dysfunctional family patterns can exist in either pattern. Dysfunction may exist in a symmetrical relationship that escalates or a complementary one that rigidifies.

The Healing Process During Family Therapy

The general goal of therapy, based upon the above theoretical outline, is clarification of family rules (Jackson and Watzlawick) and to provide a behavioral change within family members (Haley) which clarifies and makes functional the communication (Satir) (Jones, 1980).

The first task in the healing process of therapy is observation of the dysfunctional and functional family system. The therapist must assess to what degree change is possible (Greenberg, 1977). After this initial observation, the therapist's main function is to effect changes in the interactional sequence that precipitate and maintain symptoms or dysfunctional communication (behavior).

Interventions of Four Interactional Family Therapists

Several questions become important as the basis for interventions using the Interactional model of family therapy (Greenberg, 1977). What modal behavioral patterns are observable in the family? When do problems occur and with whom, and under what conditions do they get better or worsen in degree? What is the family trying to do about the problems? Would the identified patient or other family members be affected negatively or positively by modification or alleviation of the problem?

While the focus of therapy is designed to influence and manipulate family members and bring about change in Interactional patterns, this change can be brought about only by working with the totality of the surrounding systems within which the family is embedded. The aim of the therapy is to modify the context in which the family resides or in which the dysfunction is manifested. In this sense, it is the family organization in its context that is the focus for treatment.

In the section above, four family therapy theorists were examined in relation to their conceptualizations of the Interactional model of family therapy. As was evidenced in the above discussion, all family therapists differed slightly in their formulation of functional and dysfunctional families—although all could be subsumed under the Interactional approach. Following the conceptual differences, there are also therapeutic strategy differences among the four theorists. Thus, the clinical strategies of the four therapists—Jackson, Watzlawick, Haley, and Satir—will be outlined individually.

Don D. Jackson. Jackson conceptualizes the family as a homeostatic system that is held stable by the family rules governing the family. Content of communications as well as the number of persons involved in the therapy sessions are irrelevant because the therapist is looking for patterns or the process of interactions.

The therapist helps the family make clear the family rules by which they are operating. Before change is possible, the family must understand the rules by which they operate. Such an emphasis on knowledge of rules has resulted in Jackson's orientation being termed a *cognitive* approach (Foley, 1974). Such a cognitive approach, however, does not imply that Jackson explains the rules to the family. Rather, he wants them to experience the dysfunction so that the ambiguity becomes obvious.

In sum, the focus for therapy is on the family relationship structure rather than on the content of interactions. The process of interactions is dealt with, ignoring content. Historical material is irrelevant since the past is reenacted in the present because of the circular causality involved in each situation. Behavior change is more important than insight and it is much more effective to disturb the family system than to explain to family members what is going on. All family members will understand the ambiguity of the family rules as they experience them and subsequently discuss them. Techniques of intervention are used that allow the clarity or ambiguity of family rules to become evident.

Paul Watzlawick. Because of their working together closely, it is not surprising that the therapeutic strategies of Watzlawick and Jackson are similar. One difference is that Jackson generally discusses the interactions in terms of behavior while Watzlawick more frequently uses the term *communication.* Both consider behavior and communication as synonymous, however.

In *Pragmatics,* Watzlawick and Jackson start with the axiom that a therapist as outsider is capable of supplying a system with what the system itself cannot generate: a change in its own rules. To be therapeutic, communication must transcend the rules of communication that currently exist. One such type of curative communication is termed *paradoxical* and is considered to be a most powerful and complex intervention because it is a mirror image of pathological communication. What has been found to drive individuals crazy was ultimately considered to be able to drive them sane. For example, one type of a destructive form of communication is a pathological double bind. In this communication, there is a reciprocal "binding" and "trapping" of each person which results in high anxiety in each person. The more vulnerable person in the dyad can even become ill as a result of the communication. The mirror image of this type of communication is the therapeutic double bind in which the therapist "therapeutically binds" the patient so that there is a reciprocal binding and trapping that is positive.

A major theme in Watzlawick's writings is that the goal of therapy is behavior change. Several strategies are possible for reaching this goal. There are two types of change; first order change is change within a system, but the system itself does not change. Second order change occurs when there is a change in the system itself.

One strategy for producing second order change is "reframing." Reframing means to change the conceptual and emotional setting in which an event takes place (Watzlawick, Weakland, & Fisch, 1974). The frame in which the event is experienced is changed, which thereby changes the entire meaning of the event. Even if the behavior cannot be changed, perhaps the opinions about the behavior can be changed. Shakespeare is quoted to illustrate the point: "There is nothing either good or bad, but thinking makes it so."

In sum, Watzlawick is similar to Jackson in therapeutic strategies with emphasis on the immediate situation and the major goal of therapy being behavior change. The change in behavior is accomplished, not through insight, but through disturbance of everyday assumptions by which the family operates—by use of paradoxical techniques.

Jay Haley. As with Jackson and Watzlawick, Haley's emphasis is on process over the content of interactional behaviors between family members. Haley also concurs that there is little need for a detailed family history. A major goal of therapy is change in behavior which is accomplished by changing the presenting problem offered through reframing the problem and disturbing the family system rather than offering insight (Haley, 1971).

For Haley, a central issue in any relationship is who is in charge. Consequently, a control issue is present in any therapeutic relationship as well as in family relationships. Haley is influenced by the hypnotic techniques of Milton Erickson and deposits a "strategic" therapy in which it is necessary for the therapist to be in charge of the relationship (Erickson, 1971). For therapy to be successful, the therapist must be in control. A major strategy of therapy consequently involves the therapist making directives to the family.

According to Haley, there are two types of directives a therapist can give the family: those that involve telling the family what to do when you want them to follow the directive; and those that involve telling the family what to do when you do not want them to follow the directive. The first type involves telling the family to stop a certain behavior. The second type of directive involves the family's changing by rebelling.

An example of the first type of directive would be that of a mother who intrudes when a father and son are talking; the therapist might tell her to stop intruding. An example of the second type would be a marital couple who seemingly cannot stop arguing; the therapist might tell them to argue for at least 20 minutes, six times per day.

Having someone follow a directive that the therapist would like them to follow is difficult. When the patient is particularly resistant, directives which are not meant to be followed can be useful. Success of having directives followed depends upon several things, such as the power of the therapist and the importance of the behavior under concern. The high status of the therapist (power) helps and it also helps if the behavior is small. Helpful, too, is the technique of accompanying the directive by other messages—the therapist might stand up and wave his or her arms to magnify its importance.

Haley may be termed a "forceful" therapist since he emphasizes that instructions are not "suggested" but "given" and "directed" to the family. A task report is requested at a subsequent therapy session. If the instructions are not followed, the therapist emphasizes the importance of the instructions so that failure is not treated lightly. He believes in being hard on the family early in the therapy session and then later finding a way to excuse them.

In sum, those aspects of Haley that are unique are his emphasis on power and the forcefulness with which he treats the family. The therapist must develop a hierarchical relationship, with the therapist in control. The power of the therapist is what promotes cooperation by the family in changing their behavioral family patterns.

Virginia Satir. A basic difference between Satir and the other three family therapists previously discussed is that while Jackson, Watzlawick, and Haley's formulations rely heavily on a cybernetics model, Satir's work relies primarily on ego psychology, Gestalt therapy, communication theory, and role function.

Several of the therapeutic techniques used by the other three Interactional therapists are also used by Satir. For example, Satir attempts to disturb the family system in a manner similar to that of Jackson by use of the technique of relabeling and "reductio ad absurdum." Also used is prescribing the symptom, but this technique is modified by Satir in that she is more open with the family about what she is doing.

Satir's model of therapy may be characterized as a communication (verbal and non-verbal) analysis with emphasis on feeling (Jones, 1980). In functional communication, anything can be discussed and there is a congruence between the verbal and non-verbal level. A major goal in family therapy, therefore, is to assist the family toward functional communications.

A unique aspect of Satir, when compared with the other Interactional therapists, is her emphasis on a family history. She considers the family history essential to provide a framework on which to base current family patterns of behavior. While taking the history, she has the family concurrently discuss past events and current relationships.

A second unique aspect of Satir's therapy is that although she may at first disturb the family system, her main technique of therapy to clarify communications is insight. Through insight, Satir assists persons to clarify communications and distinguish how verbal and non-verbal sent and received (Satir, 1967a; 1967b).

A third unique aspect of Satir's approach is an emphasis on feelings. The principle of feelings is self-esteem, that is, self-esteem is the basic feeling that is felt. When the therapist talks to a person, the therapist must relate to the self-esteem of the person. Only then is it meaningful communication.

In sum, although Satir can be considered to follow the Interactional paradigm, her therapeutic strategies differ because emphasis is placed on insight and history material is brought into therapy. Both the communication analysis and growth aspects of Satir's model have been extended by her followers. Satir also places more emphasis on individual family members than do the other three Interactional therapists. Satir might intervene on an individual level while the other therapists would intervene on the family systems level. For Jackson, Watzlawick, and Haley, the family is the patient. For Satir, the family is the patient, but at times, interventions on an individual level (involving clarification of feelings issues) are necessary.

FAMILY THERAPY THEORY AS A NURSING THEORY: A REFORMULATION

In the following pages a reformulation of the Interactional model of family therapy as a nursing model is presented. The starting point in considering a nursing reformulation of the Interactional paradigm is consideration of what kind of theory the Interactional paradigm is, and awareness that the nursing reformulation is inductively conceptualized.

An important characteristic of the Interactional model of family therapy is that it is a practice theory (Jacox, 1974). A practice theory is one that is developed in a practice or in an applied field such as nursing, psychiatry, psychology, etc. (Jones & Diamond, 1982). The purpose of a practice theory is to guide therapeutic actions toward some desired goal of treatment. The theory assists the practitioner in selecting the most effective means for obtaining the desired therapeutic end (Wooldridge, et al., 1968). Dickoff and James (1968) have referred to this same type of theory as a situation-producing theory because it has a prescriptive element which guides the practitioner to produce situations of the kind that are considered desirable.

Because the Interactional model is a practice theory, reformulation of the model to a nursing model is easier, in that a nursing theory to guide therapeutic interactions must be a practice model. Thus, a reformulation to a nursing model need not involve a change in the basic purpose of the Interactional family therapy theory, where the basic purpose is to produce situations in which the family functioning is improved.

A second important consideration is that the nursing reformulation is inductively conceptualized, based upon the author's own experience as a practicing family therapist. When a theorist inductively conceptualizes, it means that particular phenomena or events have been observed to occur regularly in the same manner and we thus infer or conclude that this is the way in which they generally occur (Jacox, 1974).

An inductive hypothesis is a generalization based on observed relationships (Polit & Hungler, 1978). Based upon the observation of certain patterns, trends, or associations among phenomena, a tentative explanation or prediction of behavior is outlined. In the inductive reformulation of the Interactional paradigm, the author's observed associations are used to revise the prescriptive elements of the theory that guide the practitioner. The goal is to more effectively produce situations which have the desired effect, that is, to produce situations which are more therapeutic for families with which the nurse–therapist comes into contact.

In considering a reformulation of a theory from a different discipline, the overriding question becomes: what aspects of the theory can remain the same and what aspects of the theory need to be changed? At times the changes will evolve because the reformulation is a nursing theory. For example, family therapy evolved out of theoretical formulations about schizophrenia with a focus on pathology, whereas nursing as a practice discipline focuses on health promotion. At times the changes will evolve because of the author's own experience. For example, in the following pages many of the reformulations concerning the family nursing therapeutic process result from my experience in working with families over the past several years. Thus, the first type of changes are based upon the specific requirements for nursing theory and the second type are unique to the author's approach.

To address the changes of the nursing reformulation of the Interactional paradigm, an outline is presented in the following pages of the reformulation which parallels the outline above the Interactional paradigm. First presented is the unit of treatment where the major difference in the nursing reformulation is a de-emphasis on definitions involving pathology. Second is presented a comparison of definitions of family health and illness; again, the emphasis on family health rather than illness is evident. Each of these definitional changes are necessary because the reformulation is a nursing theory. Third presented is the healing process during family therapy and it is here where my inductive observations and experiences become apparent. The specific therapy procedure is organized around the nursing process using severe eclectic nursing concepts. Differences in therapy behaviors of my inductive nursing formulation versus the Interactional paradigm are outlined. Finally presented are research questions to test the empirical observations of the inductive nursing reformulation. In the Summary a digest of the major concepts of the nursing reformulation of the Interactional paradigm is presented.

THE UNIT OF TREATMENT

As mentioned previously, there are two ways in which one might consider the unit of treatment in a family therapy practice theory. First is the locus of pathology and second is delineation of who participates in the family therapy treatment. The first is an etiological issue while the second is a treatment issue.

Consideration of the locus of pathology becomes a much less important issue for a nursing family therapy model than it does for the Interactional family therapy model. Locus of pathology is a diagnostic issue and disease issue. The importance of locus of pathology in the Interactional model stems from the fact that family dynamics were considered as causative of schizophrenia. The overall purpose of a nursing model, on the other hand, is health promotion. A nursing assessment and nursing diagnosis are more salient, therefore, and are conceptualized as a family assessment. The nursing family assessment is discussed in more detail in a later section.

The second manner by which we consider unit of treatment is the question: who participates in the therapy sessions? My experience has been, consistent with the Interactional model, that it is most useful to have the entire family present for the initial family assessment and perhaps for a few sessions in which the presenting problem is discussed from each family member's point of view.

FAMILY HEALTH AND ILLNESS

The basic tenet of the Interactional paradigm is that the family is a *system* of interactive behaviors (Jones, 1980). Three types of models are generally considered when outlining nursing practice models: systems models, interaction models, and developmental models (Riehl & Roy, 1980). It is the systems models and interaction models of nursing practice which are most congruent with the Interactional model of family therapy. In each of these nursing models, the behavior of one person within the system is a reaction to and action toward another person in the system. Within the Interactional family therapy model, the individuals in the system define the family unit.

The definitions of a functional and dysfunctional family within the Interactional family therapy model and the systems models of nursing practice are congruent and similar. That is, a healthy functioning family is one in which the communications (behaviors) between individuals are clear. Each family member understands the communication of each other family member, and the family "rules" by which behaviors occur are clear. Family dysfunction occurs when, for some reason, the family rules of operation become unclear and thus the communications become unclear.

As discussed, the theory of pathology or breakdown in family functioning is less important for a nursing model of family therapy because the focus of nursing is on health promotion rather than disease or pathology (Hymovich & Barnard, 1973). Because the focus is on health, the important question is "What constitutes a healthy functional family?" This question is addressed in a variety of practice models of family focused nursing, i.e., by Miller & Janosik (1980) and Friedman (1981).

My own definition of health from working with families is quite congruent with the Interactional paradigm, that is, a healthy family is one in which the interactive behaviors are clear in meaning so that communications are clear between family members. A dysfunctional family that has progressed through therapy to a healthy state is one in which each family member understands the communicative behaviors of the other. Covert meanings to the behaviors are not implied. Likewise, the metacommunication is congruent with the verbal communication which signifies that what is "said" by the family member is congruent with what is meant.

The different theorists of the Interactional paradigm place differential emphasis on other aspects of the interactive behaviors, such as the role of *power* in relationships (Jackson, and particularly Haley) and the role of *feelings* (Satir). My experiences support the importance of both of these aspects of family relationships.

The power aspect of a relationship is important in any family dyad—whether it be a marital, parental, or sibling relationship. Also important, I think, is the fact that the power aspect is a dynamic phenomenon rather than a static one. In a marital dyad the husband may be the more powerful in relation to decisions about finances while the wife may be more powerful in relation to decisions about sex. Or, the power position may *change back and forth* in relation to disciplining the children.

Although we may assume that a parent is most frequently in a more powerful position than a child, this is not always the case. A child who is acting out and receiving negative attention by doing so is in a very powerful position vis-à-vis the parents. A common experience that I have noticed in dysfunctional families is that the child controls the marital relationship through the acting out. By having an outside focus, the husband and wife temporarily resolve their marital conflicts because most energy is focused on the acting-out child. In this manner, the child "heals" the marital relationship. In families that I have seen in therapy where the presenting problem is an acting-out child, I have not been surprised when, after the acting out decreases on the part of the child, the dysfunctional aspects of the marital relationship become evident.

The fact that the marital discord becomes evident when the child's acting-out behavior decreases also lends support for the definition of the family as a system of interactive behaviors where the identified patient is the symptom bearer for the family. The primary problem is the marital discord—the acting-out behavior of the child is merely a result of the marital discord. Empirically, I have noticed that when marital discord occurs, the symptom has to show up somewhere in the family since the family is interactive on a behavioral level. At times, the marital dysfunction shows up as individual symptoms in one of the spouses; at other times, it is displaced onto a child who is in the most vulnerable position. Thus, that person who presents as the "identified" patient is rarely the most sick person within the family. That person merely is bearing the family pathology.

The importance of feelings in any family relationship has also been supported by my inductive empirical observations. When family patterns become dysfunctional, I have noticed that family members are more apt to respond on a feeling level than on a cognitive level in relation to one another. They react to one another because they are hurt, angry, frustrated, etc. The importance of this fact for a situation producing theory is that we must assist family members to understand (both cognitively and experientially) what is happening before the situation can be changed.

Jackson and Haley place greatest emphasis on having family members experience the dysfunction while Satir focuses more on insight. My experience has been that *both* experiential insight and cognitive insight are important. At times it seems that Jackson and Haley talk as if the two types of insight are mutually exclusive. I believe that they complement each other; once the family has experienced the dysfunction it is frequently helpful to discuss the situation further to assist them to gain cognitive insight. Conversely, once the family has gained cognitive insight, it is at times helpful to create a situation whereby they experience the dysfunction.

Another aspect related to the importance of feelings in a nursing family therapy is that a focus on feelings keeps the therapist in tune with each family member. Since dysfunctional family members react to feelings, a therapist who is focused on feelings is more likely to be in sync with the family members. Such a focus makes the therapist more human and creates an atmosphere, I believe, in which a family member is less likely to be hurt.

Circular Causality. A central concept regarding family health and illness to explain empirical observations is the concept of circular causality. The notion of circular causality flies in the face of the traditional view of pathology as a causal sequence of linear events, and is, consequently, uniquely suited for a nursing theory of family therapy. The importance of circular causality is that it cuts through the enormous content presented by a family so that the basic patterns of behaviors between a husband and wife will be the same for interactions involving sex, parenting, shopping, etc. Once the pattern is recognized, it is only on that level that change can occur in a meaningful way. Change on the relationship level is what the Interactional theorists refer to as second-order change; it is a change in the family system itself.

The concept of circularity is congruent to the systems and interactional models of nursing practice. Particularly the models of King (1971; 1978) and Rogers (1970; 1978) outline a systems model of nursing practice. According to King (1971; 1978), man operates in a social system through communication in terms of perceptions that affect his health. The focus of nursing practice, then, is to develop a reciprocal interaction between nurse and patient so that the patient achieves the desired health goals. Rogers (1970; 1978) conceptualizes the life processes as unidirectional along the space–time continuum where continuous interactions between man and environment are characterized by wave patterns. The focus of nursing practice is to facilitate the patterning of unitary man and the environment to maintain and promote health and to prevent health problems. King's social system is analogous to the family so that the focus of family nursing practice is for the nurse to achieve positive interactions (i.e., clear communications) between family members. According to Rogers (1970; 1978), the focus of nursing practice is to achieve a harmonious interaction between each individual and the environment where the environment is the family.

The Healing Process During Family Therapy

Because the family therapy theory is a practice theory, the healing process or the prescriptive aspect of the theory is most crucial. It is through the therapeutic healing process that situations are produced which effect therapeutic outcomes for the family. Most important in a nursing reformulation of the Interactive paradigm is a specific description of the interventions which the nurse might conduct to produce a more therapeutic situation for a dysfunctional family. I have found that it is in the "healing process" aspect of the Interactional paradigm where the greatest modification has taken place in my day-to-day work with dysfunctional families.

In the following pages is presented a nursing formulation of the therapeutic interventions of the Interactional paradigm, based upon empirical observations and work with families. Two characteristics describe the nursing reformulation of interventions. First, they are organized around the nursing process (Yura & Walsh, 1978). Second, they are made operational sometimes in a manner similar to but at other times different from the original conceptualizations of the Interactional family therapist.

The nursing reformulation is organized around the nursing process because the nursing process is the core and essence of nursing. It is central to all nursing actions, applicable in any setting, within any frame of reference, any concept, any theory, or philosophy (Yura & Walsh, 1978). Organization of therapeutic nursing interventions around the nursing process is particularly helpful because the nursing process is flexible and adaptable to a number of variables; yet the nursing process is sufficiently structured so as to provide a base from which systematic nursing actions can proceed.

The revision presented here of the operational interventions did not result because a *nursing* theory of therapy is being conceptualized. The interventions derived from the Interactional model would be quite appropriate for a nursing reformulation. The reformulation presented here, however, is based on inductive empirical generalizations made over the years in working with dysfunctional families. Through systematic observations, I have come to conclusions regarding how interventions are best conceptualized and made operational (based on the Interactional model) and how these interventions are best implemented.

FAMILY THERAPY NURSING INTERVENTIONS

The Assessment Phase: Formulating a Nursing Diagnosis

To this point we have discussed nursing practice models within the systems framework—particularly the models of King and Roy. My own view is that a family assessment or family case history is an important part of the family therapy process and this family assessment emphasizes the developmental aspects of a nursing practice model (Riehl & Roy, 1980).

The family case history is a detailed, longitudinal account of the family systems through at least two generations. Specific cross-sectional data relevant to the identified patient's presenting problem is also included. The advantage of the family assessment is that it provides an enormous amount of data in an organized fashion so that a family nursing diagnosis is possible. At the same time it is quite therapeutic for the family. Inevitably, family members find out information about one another that was not known before (Jones, 1982).

The most important thing in conducting a family assessment is capturing both the static and dynamic aspects of the family system. The static elements include those aspects such as demographics and structural variables. The dynamic aspects, on the other hand, include the functional and dysfunctional relationship characteristics which are free flowing and constantly changing. The following family assessment tool is used as a guide to provide structure to the family assessment on which the family diagnosis is based. The family assessment tool presented here is a modification of a family assessment guide presented elsewhere (Jones, 1984). Depending upon the family structure and the presenting problem, slight modifications in use of the assessment guide are necessary.

FAMILY ASSESSMENT GUIDELINE

A. Family Structure
   1. Parents of nuclear family
   2. Children—ages and position within the family structure
   3. Personality description of each individual
   4. Level of education of family members
   5. Identifying individuals in nuclear home and outside the home
   6. Description of grandparents

B. Social Variables
    1. Socioeconomic class, educational level
    2. Religion
    3. Ethnicity
    4. Relationship of family to overall community
C. Presenting Problem
    1. Perception of the problem by each family member
    2. Perception of desired change by each family member
    3. Perception of the positive aspects of the family by each family member
    4. Perception of subsystems within the family by each family member
        a. Marital subsystem
        b. Parental subsystem
        c. Sibling subsystem
D. Behavioral interactive/communication patterns
    1. Who speaks to whom, when, and in what manner of tone
    2. Family themes and values
    3. Emotional climate
    4. Manner by which hostility and anger are expressed
E. Role-Relationships
    1. Who are the supportive family members? Under what conditions are they supportive and with whom?
    2. Who is included in the family coalitions, pairings, splits, triangles. When are these role-relationships formed?
    3. How does each person feel about his/her relationship with each other member of the family?
F. Family Developmental History
    1. Of the family in general
        a. History of the family of origin of each parent
        b. Developmental history of each child within the family
        c. History of role-relationship changes as each new family member entered the family
    2. Of the presenting problem
        a. Early behavioral symptoms of the problem
        b. Persons involved in the problem and role-relationships between them
        c. Behavioral patterns that evolved over time in relation to the presenting problem
G. Each family member's expectation in relation to therapy

Using a nursing family assessment guide and collecting a family history represents a break with the general focus of the Interactional paradigm as conceptualized in the first section of this chapter. It is only Satir who supports gathering a family history and she has placed little emphasis on it in more recent years. The contention of the Interactional theorists is that because past relationships are enacted in current relationships, there is no need for a family history. This reenactment is based upon the concept of circular causality.

As mentioned above, I endorse the concept of circular causality and believe it is one of the most important concepts in family therapy. I do not think, however, that this concept renders a family assessment useless. In this way I endorse a developmental model of nursing practice.

My inductive observations have shown that a family history can be useful. Although I agree that past relationships are enacted in the present, I find that much of the developmental history of the presenting problem is not known by many family members. Much of the information gathered in the family history is new to family members. Another useful aspect of this assessment guide is that it presents a non-threatening activity for the family as a group during a time when tension is high. By the time the family history is completed (which may take a couple of sessions), the family is much more at ease in the therapy relationship. A third useful aspect of the family assessment is that it provides the therapist with a great deal of information in a short amount of time. The family assessment allows for organization of data in a manner that gives the therapist an overall picture of the family functioning early in the therapy sessions.

A significant point to be made in the use of a family assessment is that therapeutic interventions can take place while the assessment is being conducted. At times therapists of the Interactional model talk as if all therapeutic interventions would be held back while a family assessment is done. It is crucial that the therapist keep in sync with the family so that new material evolving in the session itself (on a here-and-now basis) can be dealt with simultaneously with conducting the family assessment.

My purpose of conducting a family assessment is to formulate a nursing diagnosis (Gordon, 1982). Several nursing diagnoses are relevant to conceptualize the interactional dynamics of a family that is dysfunctional—for example, ineffective family coping, impaired communication within the family, or alterations in parenting skills within the family (Gordon, 1982). I have found it most useful to integrate the concepts of the Interactional model with the diagnoses and descriptions of the nursing diagnosis framework and, based upon this integration, to describe the family in functional and dysfunctional terms.

The Middle Phase: How, When, and What Way Would the Nurse Intervene?

The middle phase of family therapy represents the heart of therapy; it is during this time that the majority of therapeutic work is accomplished by the family (Jones, 1982). At this stage the nurse–therapist needs to be active (like the Interactional therapists), asking questions that stimulate the family to identify communication patterns, coalitions, issues, and concerns.

The goal of therapy at this stage is to help the family clarify their communications and restructure the rules and the process of rule making by which the family functions. The restructuring involves a change in coalitions among family members, emotional ties, and allegiances.

Increased autonomy for each family member is also a goal so that each member has greater independence in his or her own behavior. Satir (1967a) refers to this process as differentiation of self. I have found that greater independence between family members allows for roles within the family to become less rigid and previously hidden experiences of family members to be shared and accepted by others. Family members may begin to receive feedback, sometimes for the first time, regarding the reactions of others to their behavior (Jones, 1982). While some old interaction patterns may be highly resistant to change, the overall objective is to prepare the family to accept the change and be more willing to work to achieve its potentially positive benefits. That is, the objective is to remove the ineffective family coping patterns.

Several techniques derive from the Interactional paradigm. Most frequently, the techniques are described in a general manner; when they are described specifically, they are at times used differently by different therapists adhering to the same theoretical framework. In what follows several interactional paradigm techniques are outlined as I have used them, based on my reformulation of the Interactional paradigm.

An assumption of these techniques is that the family has the ability for self-care (Orem, 1980). This assumption is basic to the nursing model outlined by Orem (1980) which states that individuals have self-care abilities. In times of illness and crisis, the self-care abilities are such that there are self-care limitations. The focus of nursing practice is to design and control nursing systems to assist persons with self-care limitations to maximize self-care and improve health. The method by which the techniques are accomplished is through a reciprocal interaction between nurse and family to attain a relationship so that the nurse can assist the family toward their optimal self-care state (Orem, 1980). I conceptualize the self-care state on both an individual (i.e., the identified patient) and family (i.e., the system) level.

Clarification of Communications. When family members do not differentiate between the verbal and non-verbal levels of communication, a different message may be given on each level. The result is dysfunctional communication patterns. Clarification of communication means pointing out to the family or investigating with individuals their meanings on each level of communication. The nurse–therapist allows the family members to check out each other's meanings in communicating and thus allows them to send and receive accurate communications.

For example: A marital couple are in therapy for marital conflict. A central issue in the conflict is the husband's domination over the wife; he refuses to let her make any decisions on her own. The couple are discussing the possibility of the wife going to work because the children are getting older. The husband states to the wife, "You can go to work if you want—if you think you can still run the household and take care of the kids. You make the decision." The report (content) level of the communication is "Yes—go to work with my blessing." The command (nonverbal) level is "No don't go back to work since you will not be able to keep up the house and take care of the children."

Relabeling. Relabeling is an intervention which promotes second-order change, that is, the system is changed. Through relabeling, the therapist renames what seems to be dysfunctional behavior as functional and reasonable. The purpose of this intervention is to emphasize positive interpersonal feelings and behaviors between family members.

For example: A marital couple are in therapy for marital conflict. The wife wants to divorce the husband. A central issue in the marital conflict is the intrusion of the husband's mother. According to the wife, her mother-in-law intrudes into the marital system by consistently taking sides with the husband in marital struggles, by undermining positive intentions of the wife, and by telling the husband what he should do in relation to the wife. The wife also believes that the mother-in-law intrudes into the parental system by telling her how she should raise her children. During a lengthy discussion in therapy about the mother-in-law's "intrusiveness into the marriage," the therapist interjects and relabels the behavior as "caring." What previously was referred to as intrusiveness now becomes caring.

A second example is the case in which a son and father are in therapy. The presenting problem is acting-out behavior on the part of the son. The son complains constantly that the father will not allow him any freedom and that he constantly "nags" about everything. The therapist relabels the "nagging" as "protectiveness" toward the son. The relabeling takes away the negative motive for the father's behavior and labels it as positive.

Paradoxical Techniques. The paradoxical techniques of family therapy are primarily based on the Interactional paradigm. Although some therapists are reluctant to use them, I have found them an ingenious way to force a person to abandon old dysfunctional behaviors and learn new behaviors. Two paradoxical techniques that I have found useful are prescribing the symptom and reductio ad absurdum. Paradoxical techniques, in general, are directives given the family by the therapist when the therapist wants the family to resist. Through the resistance, the behavior is changed in a paradoxical manner. The therapist is telling the family—through a directive—*not* to change. At the same time, the therapist is covertly telling the family to change. All of the paradoxical techniques are based on the assumption that the family is somewhat resistant to change and will try to revert to the original homeostatic status with which they were comfortable at some earlier point in the family's history.

Prescribing the Symptom. Prescribing the symptom is a technique in which the therapist "orders" the family members (or individual) to continue and perhaps exacerbate the symptoms. The rationale for this intervention is based on the Interactional paradigm in that it "belittles" the symptom. Whereas the symptoms previously may have seemed out of anyone's control, after the therapist gives the directive, the symptoms begin to lose their mystery, autonomy, and power. They appear under the therapist's control. The family members become more conscious of the behaviors involved in the symptoms and consequently become better able to control the behaviors.

As this intervention is discussed by the Interactional therapists, the goal is behavioral insight rather than cognitive insight. The therapist wants the family member or members to "feel" the dysfunction of the behavior rather than to understand what is going on. As I previously mentioned in the theoretical material, I believe that both behavioral and cognitive insight are helpful goals for the family member(s) to achieve. After the family has experienced the symptom through a prescribing-the-symptom intervention, I find it useful to then discuss with the family what has happened to help them gain cognitive insight.

An example of this intervention is that of a marital couple engaged in non-productive fighting; the couple constantly ends up fighting in the therapy sessions. The therapist surprisingly asks them to continue fighting—both inside and outside the therapy sessions. In fact, they are told to increase the fighting. They are told to fight about the menu before eating so that they will not enjoy the food; they are to fight before having sex so that they will not enjoy the sex; they are to fight before they go to work in the morning so that the entire day will be spoiled. Such an injunction jars the continuing dysfunctional process and the marital couple rebels against the outsider's orders. They join against the therapist and refuse to fight. Through the refusal, the behavior becomes more functional.

Reductio Ad Absurdum. This technique reduces a family symptom to absurdity by having the family and therapist discuss it to a point of absurdity. As with prescribing the symptom, I find it useful to discuss the experience with the family after this intervention is used so that cognitive insight may be attained by the family.

An example of this technique involves a mother and father who are in family therapy with their acting-out, 14-year-old daughter—the identified patient. The primary disfunctional behavior involves the mother and daughter who are in constant conflict with one another. The therapist commiserates with the mother regarding the daughter's acting-out behavior. The therapist talks with her about the cross she bears, how awful it is, and about the fact that no one person can bear such a burden. Anyone else would have been completely crushed years and years ago by such behavior on the part of the daughter. The goal is to force the mother to say, "I didn't say it was that bad." The point is to show her that she is not as vulnerable as she seems. One important point with this technique that I have found is to insert an element of humor. It is important that the mother experience humor and not sarcasm. Again, I think it is essential to discuss the experience of the intervention with both the mother and daughter so that any misconceptions about the intervention can be resolved. Also, through understanding the dynamics of the dysfunctional behavior, a positive behavioral change between the mother and daughter is likely to be more permanent.

Family Sculpting. Family sculpting is a technique whereby the relationships between family members are recreated in physical space through the formation of physical tableaus. The tableaus or sculptures represent the emotional position of each family member vis-à-vis every other family member. The usefulness of this technique is that it allows for body movements to represent what may not be able to be expressed verbally.

Through family sculpting, persons use the physical space to create relationships between family members. As in paradoxical techniques, my contention is that it is essential to have the family discuss the sculpting to understand it on a cognitive level. I have the family discuss the meaning of the sculpting to each person, each person's interpretation of the sculpting, and each person's feelings about the tableaus that are created. An example of family sculpting is the Taylor family, consisting of a mother, father, and three children. The Taylor family is in therapy because of the 12-year-old daughter who wets the bed. During the fourth session the therapist introduces sculpting.

The therapist first outlines what each family member's role is in the activity, that is, the fact that each family member will play the role of his/herself while the sculptor positions each family member vis-à-vis each other family member. The guiding point for the positioning is the interpersonal and emotional relationship of the two individuals.

Following this, the therapist chooses a sculptor (who in this case is the identified patient). The therapist then instructs all family members to move out of their seats so that the sculpting activity can begin. The sculptor (the identified patient) physically arranges each family member in relation to how this person interprets the relationship between the two family members. During this time the therapist encourages the sculptor by asking questions such as: Are these two individuals close emotionally? Who is the more powerful of the two? Do they frequently smile or frown at each other? Is this relationship a peaceful one or a conflictual one?

After the physical activity is complete, the entire family talks of their agreement or disagreement with the sculptor's tableaus and their feelings about the tableaus. Each family member discusses how he/she might have sculpted the family differently and why. At times I have found it helpful to have more than one family member go through the process as described above. The most important thing is to have the family "process" the physical activity, that is, discuss meanings and feelings about the activity on a relationship level.

Focus on Here and Now. Focus on here-and-now interactions is the cornerstone for Interactional interventions as I use them. The emphasis theoretically is on circular causality and, consequently, patterns of interactions in the present situation will mirror patterns of interactions in past situations. The therapist does not look for causes of pathology but rather looks for patterns of dysfunctional interactions. Family members are directed to focus on present feelings rather than feelings associated with past relationships. Talking about present feelings arouses a much deeper emotional response in a person than talking about feelings in retrospect.

An example of focus on here-and-now interactions is the case of Mr. Thompson, a single parent, and his 14-year-old son who are in family therapy. The presenting problem is acting-out behavior by the son. During one session, the son screams at the father to leave the room. He states that he never wants to see the father again and that he wants to live with his mother. The father completely ignores the behavior and continues his discussion as if the son had said nothing. The therapist interjects, "Mr. Thompson, your son just told you to get out of the room and that he wanted to live with his mother. Yet you smiled and continued your discussion about your anger with your son. What were your feelings when your son screamed at you?"

The Termination Phase: Closure and Evaluation

A family rarely reaches a stage at which they are problem free. Also, different family members will be at different stages of independence and differentiation of self. Yet, I think that family members and the therapist get a sense of when the family is ready for termination. I have always found a formal termination session helpful since it allows the family the opportunity to share their overall experience in the therapy. Second, it provides closure for therapy. Third, and perhaps most important, it gives the family and therapist a chance to evaluate the family's ability to handle old problems as well as their effectiveness in coping with existing concerns (Jones, 1982).

I begin the termination session by having each family member discuss what he or she considered to be the aspect of family therapy which he/she has found the *most* useful and the *least* useful. It is always interesting to see the extent to which family members agree or disagree regarding useful aspects of the therapy. Family members inevitably have different reactions to the same experience.

After the discussion, I have family members talk about changes that have taken place over the course of therapy. Changes that have taken place on both an individual and family systems level are included. Those changes which I particularly emphasize involve functional interactional patterns and family rules. By discussing the interactional patterns—both functional and dysfunctional—the therapist is able to assess how successful the family therapy has been and what areas are still problems within the family system. Here I have found that family members generally agree. At times, it seems that the extent to which family members agree regarding functional and dysfunctional interactions indicates the degree of success of the therapy.

The final item on my agenda is to invite the family to return to therapy in the future if they feel the need for it. I have seen families who were out of therapy for several months or even a year who would return for a couple of sessions in time of crisis (Jones, 1982).

RESEARCH ISSUES IN NURSING FAMILY THERAPY

Two foci have been outlined in this chapter: first, the Interactional model of family therapy as originally conceptualized; second, a nursing reformulation as I conceptualize it. Presented below are several research questions and statements that are derived from the reformulation of the family therapy paradigm.

A unique aspect of family therapy is that it began as a research movement. Because clinicians were criticized for conducting family therapy sessions initially, they did so under the guise of conducting research. Throughout the more than 30 years of the family therapy movement, family therapy clinicians have attempted to refine and evaluate their therapy, using research. It is appropriate at this point, therefore, to outline research questions derived from the nursing reformulation of the Interactional paradigm. The framework for this discussion uses the typology of research described by Diers (1979). According to Diers, there are four levels of research studies: factor-searching, relation-searching, association-testing and causal/hypothesis-testing.

Factor-searching studies are designed to answer research questions that identify factors or describe phenomena (events or situations), and to determine how to categorize or conceptualize the phenomena. These studies are the most basic type. Such studies are important within a nursing reformulation of family therapy because there are many areas within family therapy which have not been adequately conceptualized or put into operation.

Factor-searching studies are descriptive and exploratory. In general, they are done when little is known about the topic or when the investigator wishes to study a subject from a unique perspective or within a unique context. Observational techniques are good methods of data collection for factor-searching studies. These methods are particularly useful to ascertain the meaning of an event from the individual's perspective (Dimond & Jones, 1983).

DESCRIPTIVE STUDIES OF FACTOR-SEARCHING

1. What are observational behaviors indicative of *dysfunctional* interactions in parental systems? What are observational behaviors indicative of *functional* interactions in parental systems?
2. What are observational behaviors indicative of a double bind situation?
3. What are observational behaviors indicative of a quid pro quo?
4. What are observational behaviors indicative of ambiguity of family rules?

A second level of research studies are relation-searching studies. These studies are undertaken when the factors (variables) are known, but their relationships are not (Diers, 1979). Like factor-searching studies, these studies are exploratory and descriptive (Dimond & Jones, 1983). Because the factors are known, operational and conceptual definitions are required. Comparisons are often made between groups of people or situations; for example, the phenomena being investigated may be examined by age categories, socioeconomic levels, marital status, or kinds of presenting problems.

DESCRIPTIVE STUDIES OF FACTOR-RELATING

1. Is there a relationship between functional family interactions and differentiation of self by each spouse?
2. Is there a relationship between functional family interactions and differentiation of self by each child in the family?
3. Are there differences between black and white families in the formation of family rules?
4. Is there a relationship between the stage in family development and rigidity of family rules?

The third level of research studies are association-testing studies. The aim of these studies is to test predicted relationships between factors (Diers, 1979). Hypotheses are tested, although cause-and-effect relationships cannot be determined. Association-testing studies rely on the natural variation of factors in a situation. No attempt is made to manipulate or change the condition of the phenomenon under study. Association-testing studies are referred to as correlational studies, which distinguishes them from purely descriptive, exploratory factor-searching and relation-searching studies (Dimond & Jones, 1983).

CORRELATIONAL STUDIES OF ASSOCIATION TESTING

1. Differentiation of self within each spouse will vary directly by degree of functional family interactions.
2. Differentiation of self within each child in a family will vary directly by degree of functional family interactions.
3. There will be a more rapid formation of family rules in families in one cultural group than in another.
4. Rigidity of family rules will be directly related to the stage in family development.

The fourth level of research studies is causal/hypothesis-testing. The purpose of these studies is to make statements about cause and effect. In these studies the factors (variables) are labeled "independent" or "dependent." The important distinction between causal/hypothesis-testing and association-testing studies is that the former requires intervention by the investigator in the form of manipulation of the independent variable. The latter are done in naturally occurring situations (Dimond & Jones, 1983). Thus, with causal/hypothesis-testing studies we can test clinical outcomes in relation to interventions. Causal/hypothesis-testing studies require control over all factors that might influence the relationship between the independent and dependent variables. Thus, the appropriate design is experimental (Dimond & Jones, 1983).

EXPERIMENTAL STUDIES OF CAUSAL/HYPOTHESIS TESTING

1. A focus on here-and-now interactions in family therapy will be more effective in promoting functional family interactions than a focus on past relationships and feelings.
2. A focus on family system level interventions will result in more functional family interactions.
3. Inclusion of all family members in family therapy will be more effective in promoting functional behaviors in an acting-out adolescent than inclusion of the marital couple only.
4. Family sculpting, compared to verbal interventions, will result in greater involvement for children in family therapy sessions.

The above questions are not exhaustive and are presented to indicate important research issues within a nursing reformulation of the Interactional paradigm. The restatement of several basic issues at different levels of research methodology is meant to show the reader how the same research question can be refined and tested with a more rigorous methodology. For example, in the first level of research studies (factor-searching), the concept of functional family interactions is used. In the second level (factor-relating), the extent to which functional interactions are associated with other concepts is explored. In the third level (association-testing), predicted relationships between functional interactions and other concepts are tested. Finally, in causal/hypothesis testing studies, specific interventions are tested to assess their influence in promoting functional family interactions.

FOUR CENTRAL COMPONENTS OF NURSING APPROACHES

- **Title of Chapter:** A Reformulation of the Interactional Approach to Family Therapy
- **Definitions**
- **Family:** A dynamic system of interacting and interlocking behaviors where all behavior is communication.
- **Family Environment:** The dynamic emotional field that surrounds the family and demands constant adaptation and change on the part of the family.
- **Family Health:** Successful adaptation to and integration of interactional-situational external social forces in the family environment. A healthy family is evidenced by clear communication between family members.
- **Therapist's Approach:** Active goal-directed involvement with the family. The goal is to clarify family communication and interactive behaviors. The process of therapy is organized around the nursing process.

REFERENCES

Bateson, G., Jackson, D. D., Haley, J., & Weakland, J. (1956). Toward a theory of schizophrenia. *Behavioral Science 1*, 251–264.

Berger, M. M. (1978). *Beyond the double bind: Communication and family systems theories and techniques with schizophrenics.* New York: Brunner/Mazel.

Dickoff, J., & James, P. (1968). Theory in practice discipline; Part I: Practice oriented theory. *Nursing Research, 17*, 415–435.

Diers, D. (1979). *Research in nursing practice.* Philadelphia: Lippincott.

Dimond, M., & Jones, S. (1983). *Chronic illness across the life span.* Norwalk, Conn.: Appleton-Century-Crofts.

Erickson, M. H. (1971). Indirect hypnotherapy of a bedwetting couple. In J. Haley (Ed.), *Changing Families: A family therapy reader* (pp. 65–68). New York: Grune & Stratton.

Fisch, R., Weakland, J., & Segal, L. (1982). *Tactics of change.* San Francisco: Jossey Bass.

Foley, V. (1974). *An introduction to family therapy.* New York: Grune & Stratton.

Friedman, M. M. (1981). *Family nursing: Theory and assessment.* New York: Appleton-Century-Crofts, 1981.

Gordon, M. (1982). *Nursing diagnosis: Process and application.* New York: McGraw-Hill.

Greenberg, G. S. (1977). The family interactional perspective: A study and examination of the work of Don D. Jackson. *Family Process, 16,* 385–412.

Haley, J. (1959). An interactional description of schizophrenia. *Psychiatry, 22,* 321–322.

Haley, J. (1963). *Strategies of psychotherapy.* New York: Grune & Stratton.

Haley, J. (1971). *Changing families.* New York: Grune & Stratton.

Haley, J. (1976a). Development of a theory: A history of a research project. In C. E. Sluzki and D. C. Ransom (Eds.), *Double bind: The foundation of the communication approach to the family* (pp. 59–104). New York: Grune & Stratton.

Haley, J. (1976b). *Problem solving therapy.* San Francisco: Jossey-Bass.

Haley, J. (1978). Ideas which handicap therapists. In M. Berger (Ed.), *Beyond the double bind* (pp. 65–82). New York: Brunner/Mazel.

Hymovich, D., & Barnard, M. (1973). *Family health care.* New York: McGraw-Hill.

Jackson, D. D. (1963). Brief comments: A suggestion for technical handling of paranoid patients. *Psychiatry, 26,* 306–307.

Jackson, D. D. (1965a). The study of the family. *Family Process, 4,* 1–20.

Jackson, D. D. (1965b). Family rules: The marital quid pro quo. *Arch Gen Psychiatry, 12,* 289–594.

Jackson, D. D. (1966). The individual and larger contexts. Paper presented at the 122nd Annual Meeting of the American Psychiatric Association, August, 1966. Atlantic City: N.J.

Jackson, D. D. (1967). Play, paradox, and people: Power and education. *Medical Opinion Review, 3,* 41–47.

Jackson, D. D. (1968). The question of family homeostasis. In D. D. Jackson (Ed.), *Communication, family, and marriage.* Palo Alto, Calif.: Science and Behavior Books.

Jacox, A. (1974). Theory construction in nursing: An overview. *Nursing Research, 23,* 4–13.

Jones, S. (1980). *Family therapy: A comparison of approaches.* Baltimore: Brady.

Jones, S. (1982). Family therapy as a psychiatric nursing intervention: An overview. *Advances in Psychiatric Mental Health Nursing, 1,* 1–7.

Jones, S. (1984). Techniques of family therapy. In S. Lego (Ed.), *The American handbook of psychiatric/mental health nursing* (pp. 224–234). Philadelphia: Lippincott.

Jones, S., & Dimond, D. (1982). Family theory and family therapy models: Comparative review with implications for nursing practice. *Journal of Psychiatric Nursing and Mental Health Services, 20,* 12–19.

King, I. M. (1971). *Toward a theory of nursing practice.* New York: Wiley.

King, I. M. (1978). Speech presented at Second Annual Nurse Educator Conference, December 6, 1978, New York.

Miller, J. R., & Janosik, E. H. (1980). *Family focused care.* New York: McGraw-Hill.

Orem, D. E. (1980). *Nursing concepts of practice* (2nd ed.). New York: McGraw-Hill.

Polit, D., & Hungler, B. (1978). *Nursing research: Principles and methods.* Philadelphia: Lippincott.

Riehl, J. P., & Roy, C. (1980). *Conceptual models for nursing practice* (2nd ed.). New York: Appleton-Century-Crofts.

Rogers, M. E. (1970). *An introduction to the theoretical basis of nursing.* Philadelphia: F. A. Davis.

Rogers, M. E. (1978). Nursing science: A science of unitary man. Supplementary materials for nursing theorists' general sessions from the Second Annual Nurse Educator Conference , December 6, 1978, New York.

Satir, V. (1967a). *Conjoint family therapy.* Palo Alto, Calif.: Science and Behavior Books.

Satir, V. (1967b). A family of angels. In J. Haley and L. Hoffman (Eds.), *Techniques of family therapy* (pp. 97–173). New York: Basic Books.

Sluzki, C. E., & Ransom, D. C. (Eds.), (1976). *Double bind: The foundation of the communicational approach to the family.* New York: Grune & Stratton.

Watzlawick, P., Beavin, J. H., & Jackson, D. D. (1967). *Pragmatics of human communication.* New York: W. W. Norton & Co., Inc.

Watzlawick, P., Weakland, J. H., & Fisch, R. (1974). *Change: Principles of problem formation and problem resolution.* New York: W. W. Norton & Co., Inc.

Watzlawick, P., & Weakland, J. H. (Eds.). (1977). The interactional view: Studies at the Mental Research Institute, Palo Alto, 1965–1974. New York: W. W. Norton & Co., Inc.

Wooldridge, P. J., et al. (1968). Behavioral sciences, social practice and the nursing profession. Cleveland: Case Western Reserve Press.

Yura, H., & Walsh, M. (1978). *The nursing process: Assessing, planning, implementing, evaluating.* New York: Appleton-Century-Crofts.

7

Beavers' Family Systems Approach: Reformulation For Nursing

Jean A. Werner-Beland

This chapter draws upon the work of Beavers (1977) for the analysis of families using a systems perspective and knowledge derived from this author's clinical experiences as a mental health nurse–therapist. This author's experential nursing knowledge is used to reformulate the work of Beavers so as to present a nursing approach to family therapy.

Borrowing from extant theories is not new and certainly is not unique to nursing (Norris, 1982). One reason for using the work of Beavers in this reformulation effort is that it is related to three general themes discussed by Norris from the 1978 work of Donaldson and Crowley. Norris (1982, p. 12) writes that these themes "express the core and scope of nursing" and are as follows:

1. Concern with the principles and laws that govern the life processes, well-being, and optimal functioning of human beings—sick or well
2. Concern with the patterning of human behavior in interaction with the environment in critical life-situations
3. Concern with the processes by which positive changes in health status are affected

Beavers (1977) identified optimal processes within family units as well as the processes that contribute to emotional functioning/dysfunctioning. Beavers' concerns are with patterns of human behavior within the family system as well as with the family-system interface with other social systems. With these primary concerns, individual dynamics and psychiatric diagnoses become secondary. Beavers' approach is thus seen as related to the concerns of nursing as explicated by Donaldson and Crowley.

By using knowledge developed by this author in practice to reformulate the approach of Beavers the nurse–therapist is assisted in the analysis of family-system problems, in the systematic collection of clinical data, in the identification of treatment strategies, and in the formulation of nursing diagnoses. This chapter is organized in the following manner. First, Beavers' view of environment, family, family health, and the role of the therapist are presented. Then through the use of two case examples the author's nursing approach to family therapy is presented along with ways in which a reformulation of Beavers' approach would assist with nursing therapy. The presentation of both the author's approach and the reformulation are centered upon the four central concepts of nursing (i.e., person, environment, health, and nursing).

ENVIRONMENT, FAMILY, FAMILY HEALTH, ROLE OF THERAPIST: BEAVERS' APPROACH

Beavers (1977) developed his approach to family therapy after examination and interpretation of data collected on families in a 7-year research project known as the Timberlawn Study (Lewis, et al., 1976). Families in this study ranged from those with one or more members who required psychiatric care to those who had no members under psychiatric care. These data led Beavers to apply general systems theory to the analysis and exploration of what transpires in families. Beavers cautioned that these data were collected on American nuclear families and that there is risk of making invalid inferences in extrapolating from the data to other cultures, subcultures, and one-parent families (Beavers, 1977).

Family-system functioning, according to Beavers (1977), ranges from healthy families (i.e., those optimal and adequate families where no member has been or is in need of psychiatric care) to severely dysfunctional families (i.e., those families in which at least one member is diagnosed as having process schizophrenia). Figure 7–1 summarizes the way in which families range from health to severe dysfunction, including the psychiatric disorders most often associated with specific levels of family dysfunction. Beavers also indicated that mixed patterns of functioning occur.

Environment

Environment for Beavers (1977) is the context in which family-system interactions occur. The nature of the environment external to the boundary of the family has either more or less impact upon the family system, depending upon the openness or closedness of the family-system boundary. In the optimal family system where there is a permeable or open system boundary, the environment is vast because family members are in frequent interaction with multiple other social systems and return to the family system with information that is analyzed and processed.

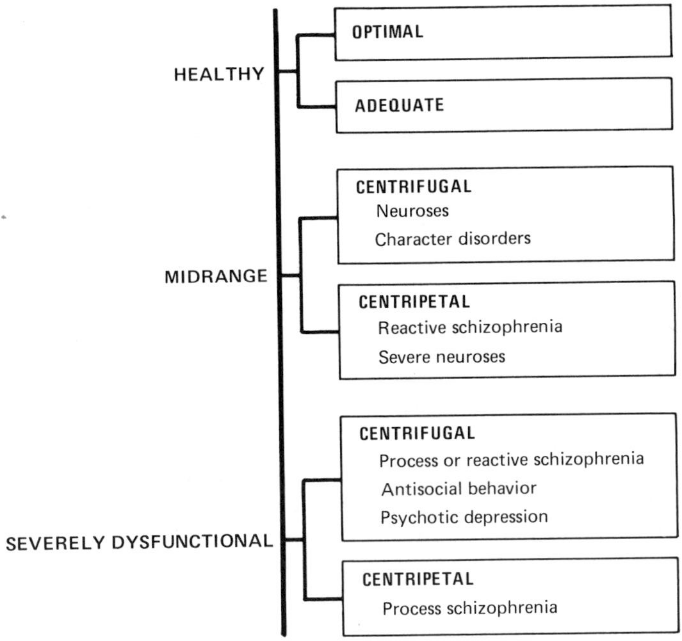

Figure 7-1. The range of family systems functioning as extrapolated from Beavers.

In midrange and severely dysfunctional families, the environment is more circumscribed because the family-system boundary is less permeable or open. In severely dysfunctional families, for example, the external world is viewed with extreme suspicion and is avoided at all costs. Environmental contact, therefore, narrows and consists of only those real or fantasized events that the family will permit to affect it or which they cannot avoid.

Family

One can infer from Beavers' writings (1977, p. 27) that a family is a system which functions as a whole to assist "the young in evolving a satisfactory identity compatible with the surrounding culture." Beavers stated a family is a system in the sense that its members interact intensely with one another and that a family boundary is created between the family and the environment.

The families Beavers studied were primarily nuclear families in which all members were related by blood or adoption. Beavers, therefore, worked with families that were homogeneous in nature (i.e., included a mother, father, and several offspring all living together under one roof).

Beavers identified eight family-system variables that are important to understand when working with families. These are summarized as:

1. *A systems orientation.* Family systems and subsystems form their view of themselves as a unit and as individuals based upon how open or closed are their system boundaries. Optimal families have the most open system boundaries of all of the family types.
2. *Boundary issues.* The healthier the system the more boundary issues are dealt with through negotiation. As systems are defined as less healthy (and more dysfunctional), system and subsystem boundaries become more closed and there is an increase in unresolvable power issues and coercion.
3. *Contextual clarity.* Healthy systems and subsystems understand and recognize quickly the meaning of communications. Communication is open and direct. In less healthy family systems there is greater clouding of issues. For example, body language is often incongruent with verbal messages.
4. *Power issues.* In healthy families power issues are minimal and parental power is shared between the parents. The less adequately a family system functions the greater is the struggle for power. Parental power is shared and parent–child role reversals are common.
5. *Encouragement of autonomy.* Healthy families encourage independence and interdependence. Each individual in the healthy family system is respected and expected to assume age-appropriate responsibilities. As family systems become more dysfunctional, members are increasingly denied individual rights and responsibilities. Subsystem boundaries become blurred.
6. *Affective issues.* Optimism and enthusiasm characterize the healthy family system. The less effective the family system is, the more the atmosphere becomes charged with pessimism, conflict, mistrust, and loss of hope.
7. *Negotiation and task performance.* Optimal families show the greatest effectiveness in problem solving and task performance. Instead of seeking input essential to problem solving, the dysfunctional family becomes more closed, and, as a result, less coherent.
8. *Transcendent values.* Healthy family systems can adapt to the changes associated with living such as aging, separation from children as they grow to adulthood, loss of loved ones through death, and even one's own death. Such changes in midrange or severely dysfunctional families produce loss of hope, helplessness, and considerable threat to whatever system integrity does exist.

These eight family-systems concepts, Beavers uses to organize the major descriptors of healthy, midrange, and severely dysfunctional families.

These concepts are also used in the nursing approach described below but are reformulated in the process.

Healthy Family

As Beavers does not define family health per se, the definition must be inferred as the opposite of Beavers' definition of emotional illness. In essence, family health or the optimal state of the system is related to a configuration of characteristics that define a healthy family. Beavers' (1977, p. 59) definition of emotional illness is:

> That condition which results from a deficiency of satisfying, coherent, self-defining experiences with meaningful others. Regardless of diagnosis, emotional illness is a deficiency disease, and one resulting from usually early failures of family–child interactions. The child is prevented from integrating the experiences necessary to provide adequate trust, self-definition, and ego skills.

Emotional health, therefore, must derive from satisfying, coherent, and self-defining experiences with meaningful others. These satisfying relationships begin early in life and continue in ways that foster the developing individual's ability to integrate experiences. The outcomes of family health may be seen in family members, that is, the outcome is trust, self-definition, and ego skills.

Although in his discussion of healthy family systems, Beavers (1977) does not define the term family health, he comments that historically mental health professionals have developed fantasized notions about what is "normal" from their observations of disturbed people. Beavers' description of a healthy family is, he stated, based upon data gathered on the most effective family systems identified for inclusion in the Timberlawn Study.

A clear understanding of the functioning of healthy families, and more specifically those families classified as optimal, is important in Beavers' view. This is so because the characteristics of the optimal family system provide the family therapist with guidelines for assessing positive change in midrange and severely dysfunctional families. It is therefore important to keep in mind that Beavers believes that there are similarities between descriptions of the optimal family and the goals that guide the practice of family therapy.

Briefly, an optimally healthy family is one that consistently supports the development of competent personalities. According to Beavers (1977), this family has permeable or open boundaries and information readily passes from the family system to other social systems and vice versa. The healthy family deals with problems through negotiation, and although its members know they are "family," they also recognize that they are individuals. Power in healthy families is age appropriate as well as appropriate to role and position within the family. The parental coalition is strong and there is a co-equal distribution of power.

The healthy family as described by Beavers encourages its members to develop autonomy. While there is a strong sense of wellness, there is also a norm that individuals are responsible for their own thoughts, feelings, and actions. In an atmosphere of openness and negotiation there develops a family system characterized by enthusiasm, empathy, and spontaneity.

Beavers' (1977) healthy family displays organized responses and accepts change. Members of such a family system can love, take risks, and accept the inevitable processes of life such as aging and loss.

In Beavers' view, family ill health or dysfunction is identified in terms of a continuum of greater and greater dysfunction as the degree of family-system entrophy increases.

Therapy

In *Psychotherapy and Growth*, Beavers (1977) briefly discusses the application of his concepts to therapeutic work with individuals and groups. He mentions that his conceptualization could be used and extended for the treatment of families. The basic notions for therapy found in his work lie in understanding the eight variables listed above.

Beavers' work (1977, pp. 23–26) suggests that one should keep in mind the following if one is to work therapeutically with family systems:

1. A family is a system composed of several individuals and is one level above the individual in terms of system complexity
2. Individuals in the family system relate to each other with greater intensity than they do to individuals outside the family boundary
3. Society is one step above the family in terms of complexity and includes many family systems within its boundaries
4. Symbolism is important in understanding an individual, a family, and larger social systems
5. All systems have boundaries that are both limiting and permeable:
   a. Too open a boundary produces a loss of system integrity and identity
   b. Too closed a boundary produces an entropic system that has a high potential for disorder
   c. A healthy system has a well-defined but permeable boundary, a high degree of orderliness, yet a potential for growth and progressive differentiation which is related to negentropy
6. Family systems have a major decision maker who provides leadership in communication with systems outside the family system. This decision maker, who may or may not be effective, helps the family system develop power and achieve goals
7. All systems require actual or symbolic space in order to grow

When individuals within a family system are identified as having emotional disorders, (regardless of what one calls the disorder) Beavers maintains that these emotional disorders: 1) are related, 2) are contextual, 3) relate to human development, 4) involve disturbances of consciousness, 5) are interactional, 6) represent a confusion of the past with the present, 7) represent a problem of effective consensual validation, 8) signify a lack of intimacy and estrangement from others, 9) include a lack of integration of individual fantasy with shared reality, 10) involve a continuing impotent/omnipotent pattern of behavior, and 11) represent a failure in obtaining and maintaining sufficient social power in close relationships. Beavers sees successful treatment of emotional disorders as requiring complete systems data which are systematically analyzed so that both the therapist and the client system can attend to these eleven points.

ENVIRONMENT, FAMILY, FAMILY HEALTH, ROLE OF THERAPIST: A NURSING VIEW

In this section several case examples are given in which Beavers' approach is reformulated using nursing knowledge derived from practice. All four concepts are implied in each case example, and at the end of the chapter the nursing view of these four concepts is made explicit. Norris (1982, p. 13) noted "because nursing is a profession, two kinds of basic concepts are required: one type related to abstract knowledge and knowing; the other type is process-oriented and answers questions about how knowledge is useful in solving nursing problems." Beavers (1977) has provided certain knowledge which is useful in describing various levels of family functioning from a systems perspective. His professional orientation, however, is psychiatry, which has a different societal mandate and purpose than nursing.

This reformulation and extension of Beavers' work is not an attempt to negate what Beavers (1977) has developed. It is, rather, an attempt to identify some of the specific differences between the approach of Beavers, and the perception of family systems concepts as seen through the eyes of a practicing mental health nurse–clinician. To accomplish this goal the concepts environment, family, healthy family, and therapy will again provide the main categories for discussion. Clinical examples will be used to illustrate and reformulate concepts.

Environment

Although Beavers (1977) pointed out the necessity of identifying the interface between the family system and the larger social system, nowhere does he imply that the therapist collect data about the family-system environment, except by discussing this with the family itself. Nursing's emphasis upon the importance of the nature of environmental influences has been evident from the time of Nightingale. Beavers' work, therefore, would be changed to reflect this environmental assessment, an assessment of the nurse as well as the family. The nursing approach to data collection is, therefore, broader than Beavers' and relies upon multiple sources outside of the family for information about their environment rather than solely on the family's perception of what it is. The nurse would visit the family at home and investigate neighborhood resources as well as deficiencies in terms of the family's needs. In addition, the nurse would contact (with the family's permission) other agencies which had dealings with the family to assess the perception of these agencies as well as their potential assistance. In all phases of family therapy the nurse–therapist is concerned with how the family views itself as a system as well as how the family relates to the world around it. The family's goals and desires would thus be identified so that these might be addressed. In all phases of therapy the nurse would use intuition and personal knowledge as well as more objective data to assess the situation.

The nurse–therapist conducts therapy sessions in the family's home if at all possible. When such an arrangement is out of the question, then one or two early sessions in the home are advisable since it is difficult to replicate typical family-system interactions when the family is outside of its own day-to-day environment. A therapist's office or a conference room places constraints on the family's response pattern and all members interact less spontaneously than in their own home. Although it is not common practice among other disciplines to conduct family therapy sessions in the home, nurses, with their orientation to home visiting as a part of community health nursing, usually consider family therapy conducted in the client system's home to be most congruent with a nursing perspective.

In the family's home the nurse herself becomes a source of information for how open or closed the family system is. Closed drapes and a protracted entrance ritual usually signify closed boundaries and a more entropic family system. Information collection in the home, therefore, and the resulting interpretations are enhanced; system boundary issues can be assessed not only in relation to the ease with which the nurse–therapist enters the family system, but also by the meaning the family attaches to the nurse–therapist's visits. The nurse reflects upon the family's perception of the visits and the impact the visits will have upon the neighbors' view of the family.

Many times families are embarrassed about having to admit the need for outside assistance with family problems. Once this initial discomfort is overcome, the nurse–therapist gathers verbal and affective cues about how much or how little a family will be willing to accept the therapy sessions. Sometimes a family will permit the nurse–therapist to physically enter the home, but will interact in such a manner that the nurse is shut out from influencing the family system's functioning. A home visit makes the contrast apparent (i.e., the nurse is welcomed into the home but the interaction during the session is less open in contrast). In this instance the door may be opened but the family-system boundary is closed to therapeutic intervention, and the home visit highlights this.

Another advantage to conducting therapy in the home is that there are many environmental cues in the home other than the actual observance of the family in interaction. These other cues aid in the assessment of the family system's orientation and include such things as: how the home appears when contrasted with other homes in the neighborhood, and the look of the home in terms of accessibility to the outside world. A case example is presented to illustrate the nursing emphasis upon environmental influences.

Case Example

A nurse–therapist visited the home of a middle-aged woman who had previously been evaluated at a psychiatric clinic. At the clinic the woman was diagnosed as suspicious and depressed, but not psychotic. She was shabbily dressed and appeared impoverished, with a low income. She was seen at the clinic as a person who had struggled so long trying to eke out an existence from substandard resources that she had abandoned all hope.

The decision of the nurse–therapist to visit this client's home was made not only because the nurse believed this a necessary part of the nursing approach, but also to assess if the family had enough resources such as food, clothing, or heat. Of course the nurse–therapist also wanted to evaluate the interaction patterns within the family system in its own environment in order to understand the nature of the problems with which the family system struggled.

The first home visit significantly altered the impressions of this woman's problems and of the family situation. The home was in a neighborhood of 30-to 40-year-old large, two-story, brick and frame houses. All of the houses in the neighborhood were well taken care of, but this woman's home was the neatest and best cared for of all. In fact, when the nurse arrived the woman's husband was carpeting the front porch and steps.

There were five children living in the home ranging in age from 13 to 19 years. Each child was neatly and stylishly dressed. The furnishings in the living room and dining room were of good quality, relatively new, and attractively arranged. In this clean, well-ordered environment sat the woman who had sought help at the clinic. She was wearing a faded, torn bathrobe, and run-down slippers. The nurse was struck by the contrast between what she expected and what she actually observed.

The initial family interview added considerably to the clarification of the family dysfunction. It was evident from the family interactions that there was little that was shared between the mother and the father. Three of the five teenagers were offspring of this parental pair and two were a niece and nephew of the father. The niece and nephew were said to be in this home because of their own chaotic home life. The teenagers in this family had little tolerance for their mother's problems, as evidenced by their interactions with her. They seemed, however, to feel guilty about her condition and were bound to the family. There was evidence, however, of their own acting-out behavior and thus their own personal turmoil.

The 17-year-old daughter had a child out of wedlock, and this 8-month-old baby lived with this daughter in the home. Everyone, yet no one specifically, seemed to have the responsibility for the care of the baby. The grandfather (the depressed woman's husband) did not take responsibility as he was too busy fixing and painting, and the woman herself was not able to attend to anyone, including herself.

It was apparent in the family session that the husband was unable to comprehend his wife's needs, and he was unaware of the seriousness of his wife's emotional state. He wondered aloud how anyone, wife or child, could have a problem when they lived in such neat, well-cared-for surroundings.

Therapeutic intervention with this family focused attention upon the interactions of the family. Attention was focused upon the polarization of parental views concerning how things should be handled. This polarization had led to considerable conflict which was unresolved and to role reversal especially between mother and female teenagers. In the therapy sessions everyone was encouraged to contribute to the identification and resolution of family problems. Some of the problems addressed were the impact of the divergent parental views on the total family, and the lack of parental subsystem boundaries to the outside world. Openness to one another was signified by more laughter and smiling. Openness to the outside world was signified by participation in church, school, and other activities.

Not infrequently the nurse–therapist will encounter families whose interactional problems are masked by their concern over real, everyday problems of living that they do not seem to know how to solve. When the nurse–therapist looks beyond the immediacy of the treatment–encounter it may become evident that the family is considerably affected by the larger environment. Oftentimes when these problems are resolved with the assistance of the nurse's environmental management interventions, the family system becomes more accessible for examination and change.

Case Example

For example, a couple in their late twenties sought family therapy because they could not cope with the many crises in their family. They had six children under the age of eight, and the mother was in her sixth month of pregnancy when the nurse–therapist made the first home visit. The 7-month-old baby had a harelip congenital deformity which worried everyone. The other children who were too young to go to school were driving their mother to distraction and she readily poured out her feelings of frustration about having six children and no time for herself. Both parents felt helpless because they had no relatives in the area and did not know who would watch their other children when it came time for the mother to deliver. The father was an hourly worker who feared he would lose his job if he took time off for maternity reasons.

The nurse–therapist first worked with the parents to accept placing the 4-year-old twins in nursery school for 4 hours each weekday, so that the mother could have some additional time when she was not involved in their care. The child with the congenital deformity was referred to a children's hospital for treatment that proved to be successful. A home-helper was arranged for so that when the mother needed to go to the hospital there would be someone who would come into the home and care for the family.

When all of these problems were dealt with the family (especially the mother, the father, and the 7-year-old daughter) focused their attention on their interpersonal problems. The parents began talking about their failures as marital partners—the wife felt she was a failure because she had had an extramarital affair, and the husband felt he was a failure because he thought it was his inadequacy that drove his wife to seek this relationship. The overall mood in the family was one of depression. The nurse–therapist discussed these issues of seeming inadequacy with the couple. In addition, she discussed their goals versus their actions in terms of the number of children they believed they could handle emotionally as well as financially. Rather than assuming some deep psychological motive, the issue was discussed directly in terms of alternatives and outcomes. The husband and wife each felt shut out by the other from shared responsibility for family functioning, and the 7-year-old daughter felt that nothing she said or did was of value. As the family explored ways to resolve their here-and-now relationship problems, the mood of the family became more optimistic and enthusiastic.

The point is that in nursing, the nurse–therapist assists families to make positive alterations in their environment. At times this may entail making necessary community contacts so as to alter the environment. The nurse–therapist will also continue to function in the conduct of face-to-face therapeutic interactions with the family. While other disciplines may identify holism as an approach to family therapy, the nurse–therapist becomes involved in this example in multiple facets of the family environment. Not only are the environmental interventions a large part of the nursing approach, but the approach is holistic in that multiple assessment categories are considered. The physical condition of family members is also taken into consideration including the way in which these might be affecting [the] family interactions. For example, the mother with the multiple pregnancies could be anemic and her fatigue and the frustration resulting from it would be an important element in the husband–wife relationship. Prenatal care of this woman would, therefore, be an important assessment category in a nursing approach to family therapy.

Family

In the practical realities of nursing therapy the family system must be considered as a whole. One cannot assume, however, that a family system adheres to the moral, legal, and ethical codes of the larger social system. Beavers' (1977) definition that "a family exists in systems terms since members' interactions with one another are relatively intense when compared to their interactions with others, creating a family boundary," is broad enough to cover a variety of possibilities (p. 27).

The nursing approach to family therapy does not judge a family as dysfunctional simply because the adult partners do not have a marriage license, or because the adult partners are of the same sex, or because there is a multigenerational system living in the home.

The important consideration in assessing any group that calls itself "family" is not only their identification that they are indeed a family but that there is some evidence of a systems' boundary that delimits the system from other systems also called "family." Napier and Whitaker (1978, p. 272), in discussing the family, stated "we do not make rigid rules about what constitutes a family. . . . Generally we start with a primary client which consists of a group of people who live under one roof." For greater clarity, however, it is helpful to this nurse–therapist to think of family as a group that not only lives under one roof, but also one whose members continually deal with the issues of Beavers' eight family-system variables, e.g., power and autonomy.

Healthy Family

Beavers (1977) writes about families being on a continuum of health, but then goes on to discuss only emotional illness or disease. This, perhaps, represents a problem that a large number of health professionals face when trying to shift their views from the medical model to a systems model for the discussion, analysis, and treatment of families. Rather than viewing optimal families as the epitome of health and severely dysfunctional families as diseased, the nursing approach presented here views the continuum as representing points that range from high-level health to low-level health. In either case the assumption is that some measure of system health is always present.

The usefulness of Beavers' (1977) descriptions of optimal families for nursing lies in the fact that the therapist uses these factors as guideposts to assess how far and in what ways a family system deviates from high-level health. Equally as important, the nurse–therapist can use these factors to assess relative degrees of health in families that are in pain and seeking therapeutic intervention to assist in the resolution of problems.

Earlier in this chapter two brief clinical examples were given. In these examples it would have been relatively easy to focus one's total attention upon the problems of these family systems. To do so, however, would severely limit the nurse–therapist's ability to work with the healthy aspects of these family systems. It is through supporting and focusing upon healthy family functioning that the nurse–therapist assists the family to change. One can infer, for example, in either of the above cases that the family boundaries are not as open as is optimal. Nevertheless, the boundaries are open, and there is health present. The healthy aspects of these systems will assist the nurse–therapist to address the boundary issues and to have access to family interactions, perceptions, and attempts at problem resolution. Once the nurse–therapist assists the family to establish more open patterns of interaction, the therapist becomes vital to the process of change.

Using Beavers' family-system variables, but modifying them with the nursing perspective discussed above, it is possible for a family-system analysis to proceed by asking, in turn, how the family demonstrates health in relation to each of Beavers' variables. What seems to block the family from a higher level of health in relation to each variable is also an assessment area. The nurse assesses the most likely avenue for change so that a higher level of health can be attained and maintained. In the nursing approach, the family's goals are vitally important and not something superimposed upon the family. In this approach the nurse would discuss with the family how much change this family is willing and needing to make. The nurse's opinions in this regard are stated as an expert's in family therapy. If, however, the descriptions of optimal families (Beavers, 1977) are accepted in toto as the only indicators of positive therapeutic outcome, much of what a nurse–therapist sees as change will fall short of these goals.

Therapy

Several suggestions for nurse–therapists have been included in the preceding sections. In the discussion of environment, the importance of the nurse–therapist's assessing and changing environmental elements was discussed. The nurse becomes a vital part of the family's environment not only through the environmental manipulations but in the changes that are addressed in the interaction patterns. The nursing approach fosters the establishment of this vital relationship through conducting therapy in the family's home whenever possible. Unlike other approaches, the nursing approach at times addresses the resolution of family problems by assisting the family to identify and use the resources of the environment outside of the family. The assumption is made that when environmental stress is minimized, problematic interactional patterns within the family system become easier to identify and change.

In the nursing approach, the family and family health as an optimal state are identified in a flexible manner. Persons living together who consider themselves to be a family are "family" even though the nurse–therapist's personal value system may define family somewhat differently. Family patterns, in terms of relative intensity, are addressed, using appropriate content from Beavers' eight family-system variables. Appropriate environmental manipulations are also made.

The nurse–therapist assesses the family system in terms of relative health. This optimistic view places the nurse in a position to assist the family to capitalize on the healthy aspects of the family system, in order to gain even greater health. The steps in therapy are those that assist the family to identify and alter interactional patterns that block the achievement of a higher level of health. The nursing approach provides options for change as well as opportunities to experience the positive effects of change. Without opportunities to experience the positive effects of change the efforts of the family and the nurse–therapist may be in vain because therapy needs to be an experiential as well as an intellectual exercise.

RESEARCH AND EVALUATION

There are many ways that the conceptualizations presented in this chapter may be examined and evaluated for practice. First, as the Beavers' variables for assessment of families in therapy was reformulated using one nurse's inductively derived nursing knowledge, the therapy outcomes of these reformulations should be examined in terms of nursing's perspective—namely the standards of practice, the Social Policy Statement, and nursing models. One might question from these perspectives if indeed the approach presented here is congruent with an overall nursing perspective. This is a valid issue whenever induction is used: Popper and Maslow, referred to in Chapter 1, have discussed the possibility of altered individual perception. It is also relatively easy to carry a simple truth beyond its limits. The nursing approach presented here might be evaluated, therefore, for congruence with other or overall nursing perspectives.

In addition, the reformulated approach presented here might be evaluated in terms of the outcomes of practice. Examination is especially crucial in this regard because Beavers' approach is not a well-tested family therapy approach. Examination of the fruitfulness of the reformulated approach is important. A large-scale study does not need to be undertaken in this regard, but certain relationships should be examined. For example, the effect upon the therapy process and outcomes of the nurse actively managing environmental factors should be examined. Is this more or less effective than those approaches which do not advocate this approach? The effect of the home as the preferred place of therapy also needs to be addressed in terms of therapy outcomes. There may very well be specific instances in which home-based therapy is more or less effective. This is an almost unknown therapy element because the research to thoroughly examine this locale element is all but nonexistent.

Finally, the therapy approach presented here should be examined in terms of the relational statements that are implied. From these statements it should be asked: Can fruitful hypotheses be derived? Are the hypotheses, once tested, supportive of an effective therapy approach? Once these types of research and practice evaluation questions have been addressed, one may ask comparative analyses questions. That is, the effectiveness of this nursing approach to other nursing approaches to family therapy may be addressed. Finally, the appropriateness of outcomes to nursing's overall goals may also be examined. Long before these steps are taken, however, the approach presented here needs to be more fully explicated. It is the hope of this author that others will examine Beavers' approach as a possibly fruitful one which may be changed as needed for nursing practice.

FOUR CENTRAL COMPONENTS OF NURSING APPROACHES

- **Title of Chapter:** Beavers' Family Systems Approach: Reformulation for Nursing
- **Definitions**
- **Family:** A social system with members who interact intensively with one another, with fluctuating boundaries which are sometimes permeable (open) to the external environment and at times less open.
- **Family Environment:** The external environment is all physical and social systems outside of the family.
- **Family Health:** An optimal state in which people in the family develop a coherence. Also a flexibility to meet subsystem growth and developmental needs as well as an openness or permeability of the family-system boundaries. The ability to change and draw upon external environment for support.
- **Therapist's Approach:** A nursing approach that takes into consideration the needs of members and the family system as a whole. The nurse–therapist assesses the family system in their home environment and manipulates environmental elements to ease stress upon and within the family system.

REFERENCES

Beavers, W. R. (1977). *Psychotherapy and growth: A family systems perspective.* New York: Brunner/Mazel.

Gordon, M. (1982). *Nursing diagnosis: Process and application.* New York: McGraw-Hill.

Lewis, J. M., Beavers, W. R., Gossett, J. T., & Phillips, V. A. (1976). *No single thread: Psychological health in family systems.* New York: Brunner/Mazel.

Napier, A. Y. & Whitaker, C. A. (1978). *The family crucible.* New York: Harper & Row.

Norris, C. M. (1982). *Concept clarification in nursing.* Rockville, Md.: Aspen Systems.

— APPROACH FOUR

Inductive Development Of a Nursing Approach To Family Therapy

8

An Inductively Derived Family Therapy Approach for Nursing

Ann M. Zuzich and Carol Boyd

The clinical practice of nursing involves immersing oneself in the client's world. Once this occurs, the nursing practice includes the sorting out of relevant facts, the drawing of conclusions, and the implementation and the evaluation of a plan of care.

Nursing's approach to family therapy involves a similar process: the nurse–therapist joins the family and immerses herself/himself in the overt messages and covert meanings of the family. Once the nurse family therapist joins the family, the nurse begins to assess the family's environment and behavior in order to experientially ground the developing therapy care plan in the meaning of the family experience.

Nursing's approach to family therapy, like the nursing process, is iterative. Family therapy, as a nursing process, involves continual assessment, planning, implementation, and evaluation. The nurse family therapist, as part of the family system, is always involved in this continuous process and the therapist's nursing skill often dictates whether the family perceives success after having engaged in the process.

Nursing family therapy, however, involves more than just understanding the steps of the nursing process. A nursing practice theory is also needed to provide the nurse family therapist with direction: direction with regards to decision making and implementation. Unfortunately, at this point in nursing's development, there are few nursing practice theories in the area of family therapy. Nurse family therapists have begun to cope with this dearth in one of two ways: first, they have used a process of deduction and deductive reformulation in order to develop nursing family therapy theory. This approach to family therapy theory building has been demonstrated in previous chapters of this book.

A second approach to building nursing theory finds its origins in the process of induction. This theory-building process involves using the nurse's years of nursing experience, and from these experiences, assumptions, propositions, and concepts are developed. It is these assumptions, propositions, and concepts that form the building blocks of an inductively developed nursing therapy theory; a theory which can eventually provide direction for nursing practice and research in the practice area of family therapy. The purpose of the following discussion is to delineate one method of inductive formulation of theory for the purpose of eventually building a family therapy theory. This chapter is divided into four sections in order to communicate this inductive process.

The first section provides the reader with the authors' views of four concepts relevant to nursing's proposed metaparadigm: family, family environment, family mental health, and nurse family therapist. The purpose of this discussion is to provide the reader with a general overview of the authors' positions on these important concepts.

The second portion of this chapter is specifically directed at the process of inductive formulation. Following a brief discussion of the components of a theory, three nursing case examples are presented. These case examples characterize one nurse family therapist's many years of experience in family therapy, and from these case examples many implicit assumptions and propositions emerge. In the past, these statements have guided this nurse's practice. Until this time, however, these statements have never been pulled together and put in writing. It is the process of conceptualizing the nurse family therapist's statements into assumptions and propositions which represents an initial step toward theory development.

The third section of this chapter involves a discussion of the induced assumptions and propositions. These statements are discussed as they relate to nursing's metaparadigm. The chapter concludes with a discussion of future research implications, particularly as these implications relate to an emerging family therapy theory.

THE FAMILY, FAMILY ENVIRONMENT, FAMILY HEALTH AND THE NURSE FAMILY THERAPIST

The Social Policy Statement is nursing's professional statement; a statement which provides a fundamental foundation to nursing practice. "The statement presents facts and values in nursing as they govern relationships to the larger professional and social context." (American Nurses Association, 1981, p. 1). Hence, the Social Policy Statement functions as a broad framework in which to define and guide nursing practice. The Social Policy Statement focuses on the social context of nursing as well as on the nature and scope of nursing practice.

The following view presented of the family, family environment, family health, and the role of the family therapist has emerged from years of combined study, clinical practice, and teaching. The theory developed here is reflective of, and consistent with, the view of individuals, families, and nursing in the Social Policy Statement (American Nurses Association, 1981). Furthermore, these family concepts are believed to be related to, but more specific than, the four concepts relevant to nursing's metaparadigm (Fawcett, 1983): person, environment, health, and nursing.

Family

The family is seen as an open system embedded in a social system. The family is treated as a primary unit, a social unit into which people are incorporated. These persons play various roles in the overall family and the optimal functioning of the family unit depends on each member's ability to accommodate and grow with changes in individual roles, the collective family role, and the society. The family environment, then, is conceptualized as the society external to the family and the society in which the family lives. The continuous evaluative changes in the family environment (society) are conceived as continually having an impact on the family system. Likewise, the family system is perceived as interacting with and changing the society in which the family is imbedded.

Family Environment

Studies outside of nursing demonstrated that the structure and function of families are heavily influenced by the society within which the family lives (Bott, 1971; Finlayson, 1976; McIntyre, 1966). In order to acquire a comprehensive data base with respect to the family, data about the physical, economic, psychological, social, and spiritual components of the environment are essential. Family therapy experience has demonstrated that dysfunctional family behaviors are very often related to environmental factors.

Family Mental Health

Evidence indicates that family mental health is a major factor in the health and well-being of individuals (Beavers, 1977). A mentally healthy family unit is seen as an effective unit, one in which the growth and developmental needs of each of the members, as well as the unit, are accommodated. The relationships within the family depend upon the balance of the communication and interaction skills of the people who compose it; this balance is reflective of the state of their mental health. The process of accommodating to growth and developmental changes is also indicative of the family mental health. Since this accommodation process is always changing, it must be continuously assessed by the family therapist. Family processes are thus a focus of the therapist's mental health assessment.

Nurse Family Therapist

The nurse family therapist builds upon nursing knowledge and experience, which includes an understanding of the process of growth and change in families. With a self-knowledge of personal values and beliefs, the nurse–therapist develops a therapeutic relationship aimed at assisting the family to maintain or improve its mental health. Thus, the nurse family therapist identifies and addresses actual and potential problems, problems which might affect the mental health of the family.

In summary, it is evident that the views presented of family, family environment, family mental health, and the role of the nurse family therapist are based on the assumption of wholeness. That is, the family is seen as an interacting system embedded within the overall environment. The family and the environment are thus interacting wholes, which are in continuous interaction. The nurse–therapist must join the family and experience the family and the environment in order to complete a valid assessment. Mentally healthy families are viewed as being able to accommodate growth and change.

AN EXPERIENTIAL APPROACH TO AN INDUCTIVE REFORMULATION OF A FAMILY THERAPY THEORY

Dubin (1978) noted that theories give one the chance to understand the relationship among the concepts upon which one focuses. A theory can be defined as a set of concepts bound together by a set of interrelated statements. It is these collective statements which allow one to make descriptions, explanations, or predictions about a phenomenon. Hardy (1974, p. 106) pointed out that the development of theory is "man's attempt to establish meaning and structure to his world." A theory then, is not developed in isolation, but rather is a cumulative, time-consuming effort by people attempting to establish the meaning of their world (Hardy, 1974).

Of particular interest here are the ideas that theories are continually evolving and that they are composed of assumptions, propositions, and concepts. Assumptions are propositions that are *assumed* to be true so as to study the consequences that follow from them. Hence, some theories consist of a basic set of assumptions (axioms), each statement independent of the other, from which propositions may later be derived (Reynolds, 1971). Establishing assumptions and the propositions related to these assumptions can be one initial approach to developing a theory. It is this approach that was used by the authors when developing an inductive family therapy theory.

Three case examples are presented below. These case examples describe one nurse's family therapy experiences with three different families. Throughout each case example nursing statements are made; these statements represent the initial foundation of an inductive, practice theory. While these statements reflect years of study, thought, and practice, these statements are not always easy to identify. Therefore, following each nursing case example, the assumptions and propositions relevant to the nurse's experiences will be summarized. A discussion of these assumptions and propositions will be presented in the next section of the chapter.

Case Example #1

This family was referred for therapy by the mother's physician. The mother recently had been discharged from a general hospital where she was treated for anemia and malnourishment. It was in the hospital that a flat affect, as well as other depressive symptoms, were identified. Information accompanying the referral showed that the father of the family was unemployed and was handicapped by the loss of both legs. There were three children: 16-year-old John, 14-year-old Elaine, and 10-year-old Elsie. John was known to have problems in school.

The house was on a street where for two blocks on one side there were a number of small industries. On the other side of the street, there were modest single-family homes, built circa 1930. Generally, the homes had front porches with small, well-kept front lawns. There was no lawn in front of this family's house, however. Instead, empty cans and papers were littered amidst the growing weeds.

Of the four steps up to the porch, two had loose, broken boards. There were broken toys under the front porch. The front window shades were drawn but clothing could be seen in a disorganized pile around the windows. The shade on the small window in the front door was completely drawn. The doorknob had been removed from the door. There was no doorbell.

When combined with behavioral observations, all of these data are significant. That the environment was reflective of, and contributing to, the woman's depressive symptoms was quite evident. A feeling of helplessness and hopelessness pervaded the family atmosphere. It is also questionable how open the family was to their environment, especially given the drawn shades and the absence of a doorknob.

The setting for the initial interview should be the family's home. The advantage of family therapy in the home has been addressed in the literature (Speck & Attneave, 1971) but whether it is more effective than office visits is still open to question. The advantages seem to outweigh the disadvantages, however, because nurse caring and nurse–family intimacy seem to be augmented when the family is in their own environment.

There is always some anxiety on the part of both the therapist and the family on the first visit. Recognition must be given to this anxiety because, unrecognized, it will affect the process of the first session. The most important goal of the first session is the establishment of a nursing relationship, hence, a caring relationship. This will reflect the therapist's belief that the family has interaction strengths, and although they are experiencing difficulty, more healthful family functioning is probable. To the degree that a professional relationship will allow, all of the nurse's skill is used to reflect and invite caring.

Since most families are referred for family therapy because there is one member of the family who is the "symptom bearer," there is often a question about the need for the therapist to see the entire family. It is necessary to be as clear as possible about this. The use of an analogy has been one method described by Smoyak (1975). In most communities, an automobile analogy is easily understood.

The family is like an automobile. Both are systems composed of many parts, organized in such a way that the purpose of the system can be achieved. The automobile is a system designed to transport persons from one place to another. The purpose of the family is not always so easy to identify.

The analogy continues by noting the similarities between the family system and the automobile system. Sometimes the automobile has a flat tire. It will still fulfill its purpose; it will transport persons. But it is much less efficient and, if it is driven, other components of the automobile system will function less efficiently and sometimes will even be destroyed. Now, the tire may be repaired or the tire may be changed, either action resulting in better functioning. After all of this, the owner discovers that a front-end alignment is needed because the car swerves on the road. The car repairs could be endless.

To relate this thinking to the family system and its parts—perhaps this family needs realignment. Perhaps this will result in effective functioning of the family system with all of its components operating at an optimal level.

The analogy sets the stage for a systems or holistic perspective. Consistent with this perspective, a useful therapy technique is to ask the family members to describe the role that they play in their family. With such an assignment, opportunities for the therapist to observe interaction processes are plentiful. As the family member identifies his/her role, encouragement is given by the therapist for the other family members to concur or disagree with the speaker. Often it is necessary to end the session before each person has had the opportunity to identify his/her role, but most of the time sufficient data will be gathered to permit the therapist to suggest some possible areas for further exploration. The stage is also set for the development of a nursing, indeed a caring, relationship.

It is important at the first session to clearly establish a contract: time, place, membership, expectations, and a method of reimbursement. The total number of sessions should also be established on that first visit. It is wise to set a date for progress evaluation so as to discuss whether therapy should continue. This sets the expectation for working sessions, while at the same time it allows for some adjustment if extra sessions seem advisable.

It is important to remember that an empathetic, caring relationship begins on the first visit and nurses learn through study and experience the techniques for beginning this relationship. Before the end of the first session, the therapist's perceptions of the family process will be shared with family members; therapeutic goals and priorities will be collaboratively established. With family agreement as to mutual goals, the therapist acts as a catalyst and facilitates new growth and further development of the family.

Case Example #1—Assumptions and their related propositions

Assumption	**Proposition**
The setting for the initial visit (interview) should be in the family's home.	Nursing care and intimacy are augmented when family is in own environment.
At first visit, anxiety is present in both therapist and family.	Therapist's recognition of own anxiety will increase family's perception of therapist's care.
Goal of first visit is to establish a caring relationship	Increased family perception of therapist's care will lead to increased therapist effectiveness in working with family problems.
The family is an open system.	Family problems become evident through a symptom bearer.

Case Example #2

The nurse–therapist had developed a relationship with the family over three sessions. The ten-year-old boy who was the symptom-bearer was identified by the teacher as having conflicted peer relationships, inattentiveness in class, and a poor academic record. There were two other boys in the family, an eight-year-old and a six-year-old. The father was a graduate engineer, employed in the automobile industry. The mother was not employed outside the home. The family had lived at the present address for 6 months.

In the past 4 years, the family had moved four times and lived in three different states. These moves were the result of the father's frequent job transfers. The house was modest and sparsely furnished and the therapist did not see a dining table.

On one visit, the boys were observed eating dinner from television trays while sitting on the floor watching television. Although this practice might demonstrate a particular cultural preference, that was not the case in this family. During the therapy sessions, the children were quiet and everyone was very well behaved. There was a constrained mood in the family;

emotional distance between all family members was evident. In order to minimize the emotional distance, the therapist suggested that, since the appointment date was scheduled for Valentine's Day, they have dinner together. The nurse family therapist said she would bring dessert. The boys were enthusiastic about the idea.

At the dinner, the mother stated it had been necessary to borrow a card table from a neighbor to use as a dining table. The boys said they were impressed that the family was eating together, not a usual practice. With the therapist acting as a catalyst, the family began to interact with one another during the meal. The process was difficult for them because of their detachment from one another.

The family meal appeared to have some potential for helping this family decrease their disengagement from one another and to increase their attachment. After further analyses, the poor academic record was seen as in part an attachment problem between the child and the school and community: a problem that reflected the family's general attachment patterns. Hence, assessment occurred on three conceptual levels: within the individual subsystem, at the interface of the individual and the family system, and at the interface of the family system with the community.

Case Example #2—Assumptions and their related propositions

Assumption	Proposition
The nurse family therapist functions as a catalyst.	If a nurse family therapist enters the family system, change in the system will occur.
Frequent changes in a family's environment constitute a family stressor.	The greater the number of family environmental changes the greater the family's stress.
Detachment can occur in a family undergoing stress.	Family detachment is probably preceded by a family stressor.
Family attachment and family detachment can be characterized on a continuum and neither pole characterizes family mental health.	Mentally healthy families are families that are balanced between attachment/detachment.

Case Example #3

The identified patient was a 15-year-old girl referred by her teacher because of poor academic performance, withdrawn social behavior, and instances of explosive anger. The family consisted of a mother, a father, and a 10-year-old brother.

At the fifth home visit, the nurse–therapist suggested taping the family therapy session so that the family could hear themselves communicating with each other. The intent was to try to assist the mother to recognize her consistent interruption of the daughter's statements. The nurse–therapist, in the previous sessions, had repeatedly identified and attempted to stop the verbal interchange so that the interruption pattern would be evident. Change in this communication pattern had not, however, resulted from this intervention.

When she heard the taped session, the mother was astonished. She had never realized that she continually finished her daughter's statements. During this session, not once had the girl been able to finish a statement without help from her mother. The mother listened to the tape more than once so that she could be absolutely sure that it was, indeed, her voice.

The use of audiotaping thus assisted this family to identify and validate a dysfunctional communication pattern. Videotaping, family sculpting, and role playing are all useful techniques to assist family members to identify their roles and interactions with each other. These techniques may assist the family to give priorities to the changes they wish to make. The role of the therapist is to assist the family in their understanding of the interaction process, using many techniques.

At times, a breakdown will occur between the interface of the family system and other larger systems. It is often the job of the nurse–therapist to support family leaders in developing more effective interactive processes. Families with school age children frequently need assistance with school systems, while families with aged members might need help with the Social Security system. Many families, regardless of their developmental level, need assistance with the health care system. Knowledge of resources, as well as ways in which families may be supported to use societal systems, is an important way to promote family effectiveness and thus better mental health.

Case Example #3—Assumptions and their related propositions

Assumption	Proposition
Family systems are characterized by dynamic communication patterns.	Using selected techniques, a nurse family therapist can change communication patterns within a family.

DISCUSSION OF ASSUMPTIONS, PROPOSITIONS WITHIN NURSING'S METAPARADIGM

Fawcett (1983, p. 11) suggests that nursing theories are sets of concepts and propositions that address nursing's metaparadigm phenomena by "specifying relations among variables derived from these phenomena." Earlier in this chapter, the concepts of family, family environment, family health, and the role of the nurse family therapist were discussed. Since these concepts are believed to be derivatives of the central concepts of nursing's metaparadigm, the previously mentioned assumptions and propositions will be discussed within the context of these four concepts. This will allow the reader to observe the consistency with which the concepts of family, family environment, family health, and the nurse family therapist relate to the assumptions and propositions mentioned in the vignettes of the hypothetical families found in the case examples.

Within this theoretical formulation, "wholeness" consistently characterizes the conceptualization of family and environment. In summary of the authors' position: family and environment are posited as open, exchanging systems that are in continuous interaction with each other. Family mental health is seen as the ability of the family unit to productively accommodate the changes in the environment as well as the changes in individuals within the family. A nurse family therapist, bringing to the family his/her nursing knowledge, assesses the family's ability to accommodate change in their communication and behavior and then establishes a therapeutic relationship in order to maintain or improve the family's ability to accommodate behavioral change. The nurse family therapist enters the family system in order to assess and change family health problems arising from family stress.

The assumptions characterized in the first case example are consistent with this discussion of family, family environment, family mental health, and nursing family therapist. These assumptions, however, with their related propositions, are specific to family therapy practice. Interestingly, three of the propositions consistently introduce the concept of care. Care is a phenomenon which is mentioned several times in the vignette.

Based on the first case example, the concept of care emerges as a concept central to a nursing focus. Other concepts related to care include family anxiety, therapist effectiveness, and symptom bearer. In the future, theoretical definitions, operational definitions, and hypotheses will need to be developed from these assumptions, propositions, and concepts.

In this example, indicators of nursing care include visiting family in their home, eating a meal with them, establishing clear roles, and treating the family as a whole. This nursing care is believed to ameliorate or improve the family condition. This example provides evidence of improvement in the family condition.

The second case example offers four more assumptions. The first two of these assumptions are consistent with the notion that family and environment are systems that continuously effect each other. The first assumption also deals with the concept of the nurse as a catalyst; this assumption implies that when another person from outside the family (from the environment) joins the family, the family will change. The second assumption addresses the impact of the environment on the family.

The other two assumptions introduce the interrelated concepts of detachment, attachment, family stress, and the relationship of these concepts to mental health. The propositions emerging from these assumptions are believed to be consistent with the focus on family as an open system as well as the characteristics of a mentally healthy family. Again, future theory development is needed in defining these concepts as well as deducing hypotheses from the propositions.

The last case example produces only one new assumption. This is not surprising because the family nurse therapist brings many of the same assumptions and propositions to each situation. If 100 case examples were studied, each one created by the same nurse, there might be only 10 assumptions in the evolving theory. Assumptions are statements of belief and generally relatively few belief statements are needed in a theory. It is the assumptions which set the stage for the theoretical propositions and the research hypotheses deduced from these propositions. As compared to assumptions, it is the propositions which have greater visibility within a theory.

The assumption from case example three is consistent with the previously mentioned conceptualizations of family and family environment and its related proposition is also consistent with the definition of family mental health. The additional concept mentioned, relative to this case example, is communication patterns. This concept hopefully will be rendered more useful when future theory development strategies are applied to it.

Table 8-1 summarizes the major assumptions, propositions, and concepts of this beginning theory. As stated earlier, this chapter offers an initial attempt at theory building, as well as an example of how inductive formulation is initiated. The summary (Table 8-1) may find additional statements missed by the authors. Nonetheless, this inductive formulation represents a first step toward a family therapy theory based on nursing experience.

FAMILY THERAPY AND THE CONCEPTS OF FAMILY, FAMILY ENVIRONMENT, NURSE FAMILY THERAPIST, AND FAMILY MENTAL HEALTH

The relationship between the major concepts mentioned in this family therapy theory, as well as the concepts of family, family environment, nurse family therapist, and family mental health are characterized in Figure 8-1. A caring nurse family therapist is seen as part of the family's environment, an environment that is capable of contributing to family stress, family communication patterns, family behavioral changes, and impaired family mental health. In this framework, the nurse family therapist functions as an environmental catalyst; a catalyst that has an impact on the family system and causes changes in communication and behavior within the system. The nurse family therapist facilitates a family

TABLE 8-1. SUMMARY OF THE EMERGING FAMILY THERAPY THEORY

Assumptions	Major Concepts	Propositions
The setting for the initial visit should be in the home	a) Care	Nursing care is augmented when family is in own environment.
At the first visit, anxiety is present in both the family and the therapist	a) Anxiety b) Care	Therapist's recognition of first visit anxiety with family's increased perception of therapist's care.
Goal of first visit is to establish a caring relationship	a) Care	Increased family perception of therapist's care will lead to increased therapist effectiveness in working with a family.
The family is an open system	a) Family open system b) Symptom bearer	Family problems become evident through a symptom bearer.
The family nurse therapist functions as a catalyst	(Nurse as) a) Catalyst	If a nurse family therapist enters a family system, change in the system will occur.
Frequent changes in the family environment constitute a family stressor. (Family system is embedded in environmental system)	a) Family environment b) Family stress	The greater the number of family environmental changes the greater the family's stress.
Detachment can occur in a family undergoing stress	a) Detachment b) Family stress	Family detachment is probably preceded by a family stressor.
Family attachment and family detachment can be characterized on a continuum with neither pole characterizing family mental health	a) Family attachment b) Family detachment c) Family mental health	Mentally healthy families are families that are balanced between attachment and detachment.
Family systems are characterized by dynamic communication patterns	a) Communication patterns	Using selected techniques, the nurse family therapist can change communication patterns within a family.

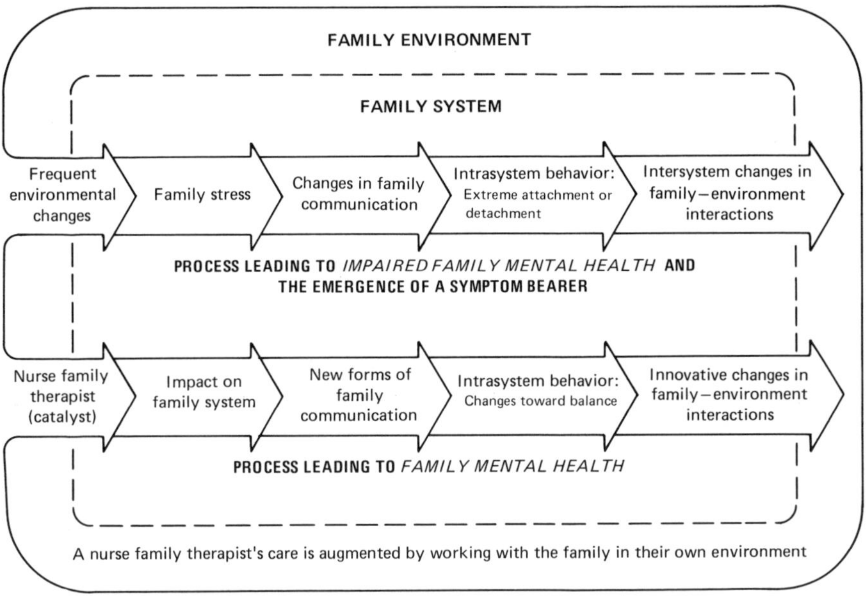

Figure 8-1. Family therapy.

process in establishing a balance between family attachment/detachment behaviors. When a balance is evident, the family is considered to engage in behaviors that are indicative of mental health.

Obviously, greater work is needed in developing this theory. Yet, despite the long road ahead, this discussion is not without value. The process of inductive formulation, a theory-building strategy which draws on years of nursing experience, allows for the development of a theory grounded in the practice needs of the nurse family therapists who use it. It is a theory-building strategy that implies that practicing nurse family therapists can make major contributions to nursing theory development.

FUTURE RESEARCH IMPLICATIONS

The theory-building strategy of inductive formulation allows the theorist to move from the experiential level to theory, rather than the more popular method of moving from theory to practice application. Before this attempt at theory building can be labelled a useful theory, however, two immediate issues need to be addressed. First, there are gaps between some of the propositions. These gaps need to be filled by other propositions consistent with, and based on, the nurse family therapist's practice. Second, there is a need for theoretical and operational definitions of the major concepts.

These definitions will also need to be consistent with the nurse family therapist's definitions of family, family environment, and family mental health as well as the nurse's assumptions and nursing practice. The operational definitions of these concepts may be particularly difficult because the theoretical definitions may not allow for an easy measure of the concept. Nonetheless, developing thoughtful definitions is a crucial step in theory building. When this is accomplished, it will be possible to logically derive testable hypotheses from the propositions.

In Chapter 6, Jones discusses the role of factor-relating research. This is considered descriptive in that these studies often attempt to relate and compare phenomena. Once testable hypotheses can be derived from inductively formulated propositions, factor-relating research can be instigated.

There are several factor-relating statements that emerge from the family therapy theory described in this chapter. These factor-relating statements include many of the major concepts mentioned earlier. It is from these statements that researchers will eventually develop hypotheses and it is the testing of these hypotheses that will enable the researcher and theorist to decide whether the data support the hypotheses, thereby lending support to the theory. Ultimately, it is through hypothesis-testing research that these propositions will find empirical support; a support that is necessary in order to move the propositions from one nurse's experience to a theory for many nurses' practices.

Examples of factor-relating statements relevant to the family therapy theory discussed earlier are listed below. These statements provide direction for future factor-relating research endeavors.

1. Is there a relationship between a nurse family therapist's care and family anxiety?
2. Is there a relationship between the number of family problems and the presence of a symptom bearer in the family?
3. Is there a relationship between the presence of a nurse family therapist and change in the family system?
4. Is there a relationship between environmental changes and family stress?
5. Is there a relationship between attachment/detachment behaviors and family stress?

SUMMARY

The family therapy theory, developed and discussed in this chapter, is consistent with nursing's Social Policy Statement (ANA, 1981), particularly in the areas of nursing's interest in health and human responses, nursing's commitment to professional specialization, and nursing's continued recognition of the importance of theory-based practice. Furthermore, this policy statement reflects the belief that nurses are guided by a philosophy of care and provide care to people in a variety of health states and in a variety of environments. All of these policy statement issues are addressed in this theory, a theory which emerged from a practice that was grounded in nursing's Social Policy Statement.

Recently, nurse theorists (Norris, 1982; Walker & Avant, 1983) have begun to provide support and direction to nurses who wish to delineate their own inductive process. Norris (1982) notes that in nursing, inductively derived theory is empirically based in the clinical situation. The theory emerges from the nurse's own clinical observations and, in turn, the observations are analyzed and used to develop pertinent propositions and concepts, concepts that will be operationally honed to help form hypotheses. This form of nursing theory always remains closely tied to its practice base.

The inductive process of building family therapy theory for nursing continues. It is a process that is grounded in experience but is not necessarily limited by it. Inductive theory-building techniques have an important place in the development of nursing science and as nurses begin to recognize their value their role in building nursing science will become greater.

FOUR CENTRAL COMPONENTS OF NURSING APPROACHES

- **Title of Chapter:** An Inductively Derived Family Therapy Approach for Nursing
- **Definitions**
- **Family:** The family is an open system embedded in a social system. The family is the primary unit, a social unit into which individuals are incorporated, and these individuals have various roles within the family unit.
- **Family Environment:** Family environment is conceptualized as the society external to the family and the society in which the family lives.
- **Family Mental Health:** A mentally healthy family unit is seen as a working unit, one in which the growth and developmental needs of each of the members, as well as the unit, are accommodated. The relationships within the family depend upon the balance of the communication and interaction skills of the individuals which compose it. This balance is reflective of the state of their mental health.
- **Therapist's Approach.** The nurse–therapist builds upon nursing knowledge and experience, which includes understanding of the process of growth and change in families. The nurse–therapist

develops a therapeutic relationship aimed at assisting the family to maintain or improve its mental health status. The nurse family therapist identifies and addresses actual or potential problems, problems which might affect the mental health of the family.

REFERENCES

American Nurses Association. (1981). *Social policy statement.* Kansas City, Missouri: American Nurses Association.

Bateson, G., Jackson, D. D., Haley, J., & Weakland, J. H. (1956). Toward a theory of schizophrenia. *Behavioral Science 1,* 251–264.

Beavers, W. R. (1977). *Psychotherapy and growth.* New York: Brunner/Mazel.

Bott, E. (1971). *Family and social network* (2nd ed.). New York: Free Press.

DeWitt, K. N. (1980). The effectiveness of family therapy: A review of outcome research. In J. G. Howells (Eds.), *Advances in family psychiatry* (Vol. 2, pp. 437–465). New York: International Universities Press.

Dubin, R. (1978). *Theory building* (rev. ed.). New York: Free Press.

Fawcett, J. (1983). Hallmarks of success in nursing theory development. In P. Chinn (Ed.), *Advances in nursing theory development.* Rockville, Md.: Aspen.

Finlayson, A. (1976). Social networks as coping resources: Lay help and consultation patterns used by women in post-infarction career. *Social Science and Medicine, 10,* 87–103.

Hardy, M. (1974). Theories: Components, development, evaluation. *Nursing Research, 23*(2), 100–107.

McIntyre, J. (1966). The structural family approach to family study. In F. I. Nye, & F. M. Berardo (Eds.), *Emerging conceptual frameworks in family analysis* (pp. 52–77). New York: Macmillan.

Norris, C. (1982). *Concept clarification in nursing.* Rockville, Md.: Aspen.

Reynolds, P. (1971). *A primer of theory construction.* Indianapolis: Bobbs-Merrill.

Smoyak, S. (1975). *The psychiatric nurse as a family therapist.* New York: Wiley.

Speck, R. V., & Attneave, C. (1971). Network therapy. In J. Haley (Ed.), *Changing families* (pp. 312–332). New York: Grune & Stratton.

Walker, L., & Avant, K. (1983). *Strategies for theory construction in nursing.* Norwalk, Conn.: Appleton-Century-Crofts.

9

Summary and Closing Thoughts

Ann L. Whall

The purpose of this text is twofold: first to present four methods by which knowledge may be developed for an advanced practice area in nursing, that of family therapy, and, secondly, to present examples of these development efforts. The rationale for developing nursing approaches to family therapy is that the world views and the societal mandates of the disciplines which have developed most of the currently existing family therapy theories are different from those of nursing.

Four methods were used to develop family therapy knowledge for nursing. These methods were: derivation of an approach from a nursing model, reformulation of an existing family therapy theory using a nursing model, reformulation using inductively developed nursing knowledge, and development of an approach using primarily inductively derived nursing knowledge. The authors were asked to focus their efforts upon the development of the concepts family, family health, family environment, and nurse–therapist. Throughout this text the emphasis has been more upon the content of the approach rather than upon the theoretical method itself; this text, however, is seen as relevant to both nursing practice and nursing theory discussions.

In reviewing this text, one is struck by the diversity which results from these four methods. Methods one and two, which used the nursing models to derive or reformulate theory, seemed to produce a more unified or internally consistent approach. That is, the translation of person, environment, health, and nursing from the nursing models, into four family therapy concepts (i.e., family, family environment, family health, and nurse as therapist) was readily accomplished. This is probably because well-developed nursing models were available for these efforts and these models currently explicate the four central concepts of nursing. These concepts were readily translated into the four family therapy concepts. The task of identifying the four family therapy concepts when the inductive or inductive reformulation methods were used was more formidable. This was undoubtedly because the nursing knowledge used was not a well-developed model.

The product of the four methods differed in other ways. The first two methods which used the nursing models, although more consistent in concepts, were in some instances less specific in terms of directives for the practice. Using the more global concepts and relationships found in nursing models to derive a family therapy approach at times was very difficult. As this effort to develop nursing knowledge in the area of family therapy continues, these difficulties will not be considered insurmountable or unusual.

How is the practitioner to use the approaches found in this text? This could be addressed in several ways, and here are a few. After perusal of each of the chapters, if in the opinion of the practitioner one of the approaches appears to address issues and relationships that are thought to be important in family therapy, this approach might be examined in a specific family therapy situation. One of the more productive ways to examine the usefulness of an approach is through retrospective analysis of an actual family therapy case. Questions should be asked, such as: would the assessment suggested by the approach have yielded useful and important data in this case? would the nursing diagnosis suggested by the approach have identified major problem areas? what interventions would have been suggested by the approach? what outcomes would these interventions have most likely yielded? how would the approach have differed from the assessment, diagnosis, intervention, and outcomes of the approach which was used? In essence, these questions ask what are the pros and cons of the approach which was used versus the approach found in this text. Such examination will identify for the practitioner the major strengths and weaknesses of the selected approach as well as ways in which the nursing approach may be further developed.

Another way in which the nurse–practitioner might use the approaches presented is to ask these same questions in an ongoing family therapy situation. The nurse–therapist might examine the assessment, diagnosis, intervention, and outcomes which would be suggested by an approach found in this text versus that of the therapy approach that the practitioner usually would use. Both of these comparative analysis methods should suggest the value of the approach presented as well as ways in which this approach might be further developed. Once further development has taken place, the testing of these approaches both in clinical practice and through research should occur.

The further explication and revision of approaches presented may also be addressed by those familiar with the processes of theory development.

In the family therapy approaches presented here, the authors were asked to develop the nursing approach through explication of the concepts: family, family health, family environment, and nurse–therapist. This focus upon four concepts was seen as appropriate for a first step in theory development. The next steps must include, however, the development of other concepts specific to one approach as well as the identification of relational statements. Various methods of theory development might also be used, such as statement synthesis and analysis (Walker & Avant, 1983). As these nursing approaches are further developed, analysis and evaluation should follow these efforts, using, for example, one of the theory analysis and evaluation frameworks such as that of Fitzpatrick (Fitzpatrick & Whall, 1983). The analysis and evaluation of the approach would identify gaps and inconsistencies which might be addressed in further development efforts. Development of specific theoretical approaches, in the view presented here, is a multi-stage effort.

This discussion of the theory development efforts that are needed should not dissuade the practitioner from current examination of the approaches presented in this text in practice. It is very important that clinical insight and evidence be combined with, and stimulate these development efforts, especially when the approach to be developed is to guide clinical practice with various cultural groups.

This text presents four methods by which nursing knowledge may be developed for an advanced practice area in nursing. The four methods presented are seen as potential ways of developing the theoretical base which is needed for nursing to specifically carry out societal mandates. Certainly there are other methods by which knowledge may be developed to guide nursing approaches to family therapy. Those presented here, however, are seen as having an exciting potential to assist in the development of that distinct body of nursing knowledge which is essential to the discipline of nursing.

REFERENCES

Fitzpatrick, J., & Whall, A. (1983). *Conceptual models of nursing: Analysis and application.* Bowie, Md.: Brady.

Walker, L., & Avant, K. (1983). *Strategies for theory construction in nursing.* Norwalk, Conn.: Appleton-Century-Crofts.

Index

A

B

E

F

G

H

I

J

K

L

M

N

R

S

T

V

W

Y